# Ageless Skin Obsession

# Ageless Skin Obsession

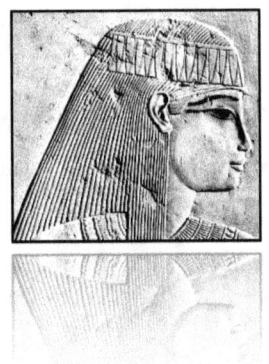

by

## Dr. Farid Mostamand

ISBN–10: 146637845X

ISBN–13: 978–1466378452

# CONTENTS

# THE EFFECT OF HOLLYWOOD, THE MEDIA AND MODELS ON AGELESS SKIN AND LOOKING YOUTHFUL

It is no secret that mainstream America is obsessed with looking good, In modern-day America, that means looking *young*, as is apparent every time we go to a movie. The actors are displayed up close and personal on ever-larger screens and in digital images that reveal every single flaw, line, and wrinkle—or, more often than not, a perfectly unlined face. When a nearly flawless-looking actor in her fifties appears on the large screen, it's obvious that some anti-aging work has taken place. The need to look young has taken America by storm, with millions of Americans working hard and spending vast amounts of money not to look their age. And why not put off wrinkles and sagging as long as possible? We are being directly or indirectly inundated by the media telling us that we should look our best all the time, looking younger means feeling better about ourselves.

"Younger is better" is the message being communicated by the models in magazines and on television; but how do these paragons of beauty achieve such perfection, and what impact does all this pressure for perfection have on the average person's self-image?

America has armies of everyday people begging to be dipped into the same fountain of youth that has kept their favorite celebrities eternally young. It is no wonder that people of all ages (from septuagenarians to teens) consider their TV and movie idols the epitome of human beauty—examples they want emulate. We see celebrity faces and bodies everywhere; in theaters, on television, in magazines and on billboards, and they leave people, particularly those from the Baby Boomer generation, thinking that is how they should look, too.

If you were to stand outside the offices of any well-known plastic surgeon's office in the Hollywood area, you would undoubtedly find photographers and paparazzi lying in wait to catch a celebrity walking in or out.

More often than not, though, what they find are everyday people with average incomes trying to capture a look they've seen in a magazine or at the movie theater.

Television shows such as Extreme Makeover and The Swan actually encourage main-stream Americans to do everything in their power to look younger and more physically attractive.

Many of today's celebrities take advantage of cosmetic procedures in order to look their best and to ensure that they stay in the limelight. The media, casting directors, photographers, and reporters all focus their attention on how celebrities look. They speculate on the negative to arouse interest. They question whether or not wrinkles have begun cropping up on Jennifer Anniston's face, and whether Madonna looks as toned as ever or if her face is beginning to sag. The men aren't immune to this scrutiny, either. They ask readers if Richard Gere looks his age or if people think he has had work done.

Veteran actors and models constantly seek ways to maintain ageless-looking skin. Christie Brinkley, an extremely successful model now close to sixty years old, works hard to stay in good physical shape, but is it any wonder that she may have had eyelid surgery to subtract a few years from her appearance? It seems that the media and the public demand that their idols stay young. They gossip about them and circulate any unflattering photos that come to light. Actress Courtney Cox has admitted publicly to taking steps to slow down the aging process by way of Botox injections, and Jennifer Anniston has confessed to rhinoplasty (a nose job).

Both young rising stars and older, more established celebrities are either having surgical procedures to fight the signs of aging or are opting for less invasive, non-surgical treatments. They are under constant scrutiny from the media; and the Hollywood community is quick to criticize if their look is less than perfect. Yet even as the media drives its stars to plastic surgery, it also criticizes those who appear to have altered themselves. Even stars as young as 24-year old Megan Fox have found themselves targeted on social media networks for having Botox injections. Ms Fox went as far as placing a recent photograph showing herself furrowing her brows on her Facebook page to dispel Botox rumors. Gossip magazines and the paparazzi seem to demand natural eternal youth.

Plastic surgeons are in great demand. They are supplying celebrities and the general public with total face lifts, stem cell and fat grafts, and other procedures that are often painful and require long recovery times, and there is always a risk that these surgical options will produce uneven or "plastic" looking results. Think of Michael Jackson's unfortunate facial surgeries; and consider whether Joan Rivers really has the face of a woman in her 70s.

Instead of going the route of plastic surgery, many Baby Boomers are opting for less drastic ways to turn back the clock. Many are flocking to dermatologists to investigate prescription skincare products that will prevent wrinkles and sagging skin. Although the media seems to steer us toward extreme solutions, most people would prefer not to undergo painful, expensive surgeries.

The market for non-surgical approaches—those that achieve the same effects without using invasive procedures—is growing rapidly, and anti-aging skincare is at the forefront of available choices.

Dermatologists are aware that their patients want to look younger without taking extreme measures. As such, many of them offer high-quality, prescription skincare lines. With so many effective in-office, non-surgical procedures such as Botox injections, laser treatment, dermal fills, and chemical peels, there is no need for surgery. Instead, skincare creams containing stem cells, peptides, collagen, and exfoliators are now used to stave off the signs of aging.

People wishing to look younger are discovering the benefits of skin lighteners, toners, hyaluronic acid, liposomes, peptides, and retinol—which are just some of the skincare products and ingredients that are relatively new to the anti-aging market. These skincare products are well worth investigating, because the more you know about them and the ingredients they contain, the more informed you will be when deciding on the best anti-aging regimen for your skin.

# ෫ 1 ൲

# UNDERSTANDING SKIN LAYERS

I n this chapter, we discuss some of the functions of the skin's layers. Once you understand how the different layers of the skin work, you can determine how to treat the skin conditions related to each layer, particularly those related to wrinkles and aging.

## Stratum Corneum

The stratum corneum is the outermost layer of skin, the last of the epidermal layers. This layer of skin is made up of dead, smooth skin cells that shed approximately every couple of weeks and are then renewed. The main function of the stratum corneum is to work as the skin's outer barrier, keeping water out and shaping the appearance of the skin by adding strength and elasticity. This layer is strong, able to absorb and release energy, and elastic, so it can hold its shape and resist any forced change.

The stratum corneum is made up of a keratin protein filament network and lipids, forming five connected layers that interact with one another. When this functional network is disrupted, as happens when we age, we see an increase in dry skin, atopic dermatitis, psoriasis, or other skin conditions.

## Epidermis

The epidermis is the most superficial of the skin's layers. It is composed of the five layers, including the stratum corneum. The bottom, or basal layer, produces the keratin by which dead skin cells are replaced on the upper layers. It takes two weeks for the new cells to move to the top layer of skin. Melanin is found in the basal epidermal layer.

The second layer is the stratum spinosum or the prickly layer. It is held together by *prickly* cells and is where protein (keratin) is synthesized. The next layer is the granular layer where melanocytes, precursors to keratin, are found. The stratum lucidum is the fourth layer, which is very thin. It is found almost exclusively in the palms of the hand and soles of the feet.

## Dermis

The dermis is the skin that lies below the epidermal layers. It is comprised of two layers: the papillary and the reticular layers. The papillary layer is composed of connective tissue, collagen, and elastin. The reticular layer contains thick connective tissue and collagen fibers. Collagen fibers are very strong and give the skin its durability and toughness. Elastin fibers keep the skin flexible and pliable. The dermis also contains hair follicles, sweat and sebaceous glands, blood vessels and fibroblasts. Fibroblasts are an integral part of the skin's structure. They produce collagen and deposit it where it is needed for growth and additional strength in the dermis. Loss of dermis can cause the epidermis to atrophy, leaving the skin thinner and more wrinkled.

## Subcutaneous Tissue – Hypodermis

The subcutaneous layer is located just below the dermis. It is a layer of fat also known as subcutaneous tissue or the hypodermis. It is made up of loose connective and adipose tissue. The hypodermis aids in metabolism and insulates the skin. Inflammation in the hypodermis can cause skin dimpling or cellulitis.

## ❖ BASIC FUNDAMENTALS FOR FLAWLESS SKIN

If we believe what we see in movies and on television, we should all have flawless skin. With their glowing, youthful looks, movie stars continue to dazzle us no matter their age, and audiences—young and old—strive to emulate them. You may have already discovered that keeping that young-looking skin is not easy unless you work hard at it and begin taking care of your skin when you are young.

### Learning to Care for Your Skin Early

The onslaught of reality TV has actually encouraged children and teenagers to start a beauty regimen early in life. With manicures and pedicures, trips to the tanning salon and facials becoming the norm before they turn thirteen, this generation is learning early that to get ahead they need to keep themselves looking their best and "putting their best foot forward." In the process, they are learning that good skincare is the only way to achieve flawless skin.

### Start with the Basics

Regardless of your age, develop a skincare regimen that you follow daily. This should be based on your skin type and the routine should be one that will keep your skin hydrated and refreshed. This regimen should include a thorough cleansing twice a day followed by the application of a toner to restore the skin's natural pH balance. A good moisturizer should also be used daily, and if your skin tends to be dry or very sensitive, make sure that you use products that won't dry your skin further.

Sunscreen is an essential that should be used prior to any exposure to the sun's harmful UVA and UVB rays. If you spend a lot of time in the sun or outdoors, use a sunscreen with a broad spectrum of coverage (such as SPF 30 or more). Sunscreen should be reapplied after swimming or excessive perspiration and throughout the day as needed.

A weekly routine of exfoliation will keep your skin refreshed and remove any dead or dull skin cells so that new ones can be generated. Facials are a great way to rehydrate the skin on the face and neck. Schedule one on a monthly basis to keep your skin looking fresh at all times. Start using anti-wrinkle creams at an early age to combat any visible signs of premature aging. They will keep your skin nourished and full of vitality.

## Beware of Some Bad Habits

Starting your campaign for flawless skin early is great, but it is also important not to establish any bad habits that may be hard to break and that might even damage your skin. Tanning salons are all the rage right now because people want that healthy, tanned look, but if you don't use sunscreen, excessive use of artificial sun is just as bad as being exposed to the harmful UVA and UVB rays of the sun itself. Don't fall into the trap of thinking that fake tans are safe. Your skin needs protection from artificial tanning *and* from the sun in order to avoid damage that will affect your skin later in life.

It is essential that you understand your skin type if you want to ensure that the skincare products you use are appropriate. Many products can dry the skin or irritate it without your knowledge. These products may defeat your whole strategy for keeping your skin looking flawless.

Seek advice from a dermatologist if your skin is prone to acne or blemishes or if you have conditions like rosacea or eczema, as those conditions may influence the type of products that you should choose.

## ❖ IT IS NEVER TOO EARLY TO START AN ANTI-WRINKLE CAMPAIGN

Most people have seen ads for anti-wrinkle products. It is easy to say, "Well, I'm only 25 or 35, so why do I need to start using these products?", but some would argue it is never too early to begin to prepare your skin for aging and keeping those dreaded wrinkles away. These people would be right. Prevention is the best policy, especially when it comes to wrinkles. Start doing preventative maintenance now to guard against an early onslaught of wrinkles.

### The 20s are for Prevention

During the twenties, your skin might be prone to blemishes or acne, so treating these conditions correctly will prevent skin damage and premature aging from discoloration or scaring. During your 20s, you are likely to spend a lot of time in the sun, and preventing damage caused by the sun's deadly UV rays is essential if you want to keep your skin from becoming overly dry.

Here are some tips:

❖ Keep your skin clean and toned at all times. If your skin tends to be oily or acne-prone, use a cleanser and toner specifically intended for those conditions.

❖ Use a sunscreen any time you are exposed to the sun. Get into the habit of automatically using one before going out. Make sure that any exposed skin is protected against the harmful rays that can prematurely damage the skin.

❖ Keep the skin moisturized so that it is properly balanced and well hydrated. Many anti-aging products contain both moisturizers and sunscreens, so if you spend a lot of time in the sun, look for one of these multi-purpose products to prevent wrinkles and fine lines while protecting yourself from the sun's rays.

## Expand Your Anti-Aging Products in the 30s to Continue Prevention

As you reach your 30s, your skin starts to age, so it is important to keep up the regimen you began in your 20s, adding a lotion that is specifically for firming. Some of these products can be used in conjunction with your face cream. You may also want to start using something to prevent crow's feet and other fine lines around the eyes. Your 30s regimen will then be:

❖ Cleanse and tone the skin with a product appropriate for your skin type. Use products specifically for those with dry or sensitive skin or for oily skin prone to acne.

❖ Use a sunscreen during the day and replenish it as often as necessary.

❖ Keep skin moisturized and balanced, and if skin tends to be dry, use special products that will address this and keep it hydrated.

❖ Add anti-wrinkle lotion for the face and also a product made specifically for use around the eyes.

❖ Schedule a regular face mask or peel to ensure the skin is thoroughly cleansed and old skin is exfoliated to pave the way for fresh skin cells.

## Those Over 40 Require Special Anti-Aging Products

Once you reach your 40s, your skin starts to lose its youthful bloom, so it is essential to target specific areas of the skin that are prone to expression lines, crow's feet, brown spots, and other visible signs of aging. The older you get, the more care is required to keep your skin looking its best. There are many essential vitamins and minerals that are becoming depleted in the skin that need to be restored, repaired, or revitalized to keep the skin looking fresh, so in your 40s and beyond use anti-aging creams during the day and at night. These creams are to keep the skin soft and supple so that the signs of aging, like wrinkles and fine lines, are diminished.

For some people, age spots, brown spots, freckles, and other hyper-pigmentation problems can worsen as they age. If you notice these types of problems, seek products that specifically combat the spots and help even out skin tones.

If you suffer from dark circles under the eyes, there are special treatments to lighten these areas and reduce puffiness and other aging signs around the eyes.

## Pampering Your Skin after 50 Provides Youthful Results

As you age, your skin ages with you. If you don't take care of it and ensure that it is nurtured and properly protected, it can age more rapidly than normal. Because of its constant exposure to environmental stressors and harmful UV rays, the skin may lose its youthful look too soon. Outside influences and hormonal changes cause your skin to lose its elasticity and suppleness so that it is no longer as firm and taut as you would like it to be. You need to take deliberate steps to keep it replenished and looking youthful.

After 50, it is especially important to practice anti-aging skincare, particularly on the face and neck, to ensure that this fragile skin keeps its vibrant, youthful radiance as long as possible. There are ways to keep your skin healthier and younger-looking without a lot of effort on your part, and these techniques can do a world of good in helping you maintain a more youthful appearance. Pampering your skin is all about good basic care and the addition of a few extra steps. Here are some important ways that those of you over 50 can pamper yourself at home as part of your daily skincare regimen.

❖ Cleanse your skin regularly. This is a fundamental step in keeping your skin looking and feeling more youthful.

❖ Always use a cleanser that won't dehydrate the skin. Instead, use one that replenishes and moisturizes it. If your skin is sensitive or tends to be prone to rosacea, acne, and blemishes; select a cleanser specifically formulated to address these issues.

❖ Likewise, if your skin is oily, you should use a cleanser made to balance the skin and keep it hydrated while controlling the oil. Be sure to choose a gentle cleanser that won't irritate already sensitive or inflamed skin.

❖ Exfoliate to keep your skin healthy. Exfoliation should be done on a regular basis as part of your skincare regimen. It will remove sebum and dead skin cells and unclog and reduce large pores. This process is very beneficial for people who have acne or are prone to blemishes. For sensitive skin, use a gentle exfoliate that won't irritate the skin. There are facial scrubs and body scrubs that can be used regularly.

❖ Protect the Skin. This is extremely important as UVA and UVB sun rays are very damaging. They can cause premature aging as well as hyper-pigmentation and other unhealthy conditions including cancer. A sunscreen with an SPF of 15 or higher is an essential part of your skincare regimen and should be applied before any exposure to the sun. It should be reapplied as necessary throughout the day depending on your activities.

❖ Moisturize! Moisturize! Moisturize! As we age, our skin tends to become dry and more sensitive, especially in women going through menopause. Moisturizer is vital for your face and your body to ensure that the skin is constantly nourished and replenished. Left unattended, dry skin can become itchy, irritated, and red—and whether it's on the face or on your hands or feet, it is always unattractive. Dry skin can be caused by more than stress or climatic factors. It may be the soap you are using or some of the household products you use. Try switching to a gentle soap to see if it makes a difference, and use gloves to keep your skin from coming in contact with the harsh chemicals in cleaning products or, better yet, experiment with natural products to avoid the chemicals altogether. Be sure to use a good moisturizer twice daily to add moisture to the skin's surface.

Pampering your skin is an excellent way to keep it looking attractive, feeling smoother and softer, give it a better texture, and help it retain its youthful glow. Wrinkle creams and other special products used in concert with the four pampering tips for younger skin after 50 (cleanse, exfoliate, protect, and moisturize) will help you combat the aging process by reducing puffiness and dark circles under the eyes.

Here are some of the products recommended for 50-plus skincare.

## Ageless Derma Stem Cell and Peptide Anti-Wrinkle Cream

This is a revolutionary new product designed to revitalize your skin and protect it from the signs of aging. Combining seven natural, scientifically proven anti-aging ingredients into one product, Ageless Derma Stem Cell and Peptide Anti-Wrinkle Cream eliminates the appearance of fine lines and wrinkles, improves the firmness and elasticity of skin, removes crow's feet and re-energizes skin for a smoother, firmer, and younger look.

## Babors HSR Lifting Cream

Babors HSR Lifting Cream diminishes wrinkles, decreases the signs of aging, and erases fine lines by supplementing the skin's natural elastin. Babors HSR Lifting Cream is a specially formulated treatment designed to improve elasticity and delay light-induced aging.

## Physicians Complex Tissue Growth Factor

Users will achieve an unprecedented level of wrinkle reduction with the Physicians Complex Tissue Growth Factor. This product is a high-potency combination of peptides, olive oil, homeostatine, coenzyme Q-10, soy proteins, coconut endosperm, and tissue growth factors.

## DDF Advanced Firming Cream 1.7oz

DDF Advanced Firming Cream works below the skin's surface to improve hydration and increase firmness.

Able to lock in vital moisturizing elements, DDF Advanced Firming Cream is a highly advanced formula infused with a breakthrough turmeric complex that protects the skin from harmful free radical damage. Free radicals attack the moisture barriers of the skin and contribute to premature aging. DDF Advanced Firming Cream helps to reverse these effects as it instantly tightens and firms the skin from within. DDF Advanced Firming Cream should be used as part of a comprehensive, daily skincare routine.

## ◈ WRINKLES MAY SHOW MATURITY, BUT MOST PEOPLE DON'T WANT THEM

When our skin ages faster than we do, chronologically, it's called premature aging. Premature aging manifests itself as wrinkles around the eyes and mouth and as deepened expression lines. Many of these fine lines and wrinkles are hereditary, but heredity is not destiny, and much of this damage could have been prevented if proper skincare precautions had been taken.

## Aging and Wrinkles

Skin becomes thinner with age and loses its ability to retain moisture, making it dry. At the same time, aging reduces the production of collagen and elastin, which are responsible for keeping the skin firm and elastic so that it snaps back into shape when stretched. When these elements break down, the skin loses its ability to repair itself, so there is a vicious cycle of skin sagging and wrinkling as it dries out. The cycle continues unless we intervene to repair and rejuvenate our skin.

## Sun Exposure is a Major Cause of Wrinkles

One of the main causes of wrinkles, other than aging, is sunlight. Many of us grew up without knowing how harmful the sun could be or that people with fair or light skin were even more susceptible to the sun's rays than others. We spent endless hours soaking up the sun with little or no sunscreen so that our bodies were unnecessarily exposed to the UVA and UVB rays that at the very least can cause premature aging—and could potentially cause skin cancer as well.

Photo-aging occurs when there is skin damage from the sun. It is usually prevalent on the most exposed parts of the body (e.g., the face). It creates wrinkles, fine lines, sagging skin, and skin keratosis or liver spots, along with really rough, dry skin. Continued exposure over time makes the skin especially vulnerable to photo-aging if steps are not taken to prevent further damage.

## Sunscreen and the New Government Guidelines

Very recently the Federal Drug Administration (FDA) and the U.S. Government changed the guidelines regulating sunscreen products.

For the first time in over thirty years, the FDA has submitted new guidelines for the use of sunscreen products. Consumers will start to see changes on the labels of these products by the summer of 2012. If the product does not protect the user from both Ultraviolet A (UVA) and Ultraviolet B (UVB) radiation, **the label cannot state that the sunscreen protects against skin cancer or premature aging**.

Sunscreens will no longer be allowed to advertize sun protection factors (SPF) above 50. Instead, the label can only indicate that the SPF is 50+, since there is no evidence to demonstrate that protection is improved above 50 SPF.

In order to be considered a broad spectrum sun protectant, a product has to provide both UVA and UVB protection. At present, UVB protection is displayed on most sunscreen or sun block products. UVB rays can cause cancer, aging, and sun damage, but UVB rays can be blocked—by the windows in your home or the windshield in your car—because they cannot penetrate as deeply as UVA rays. UVA rays *do* penetrate and *do* cause skin damage, and both types of sunrays can cause cancer. The FDA has therefore determined that sunscreen products must protect against both.

Another change is that products will no longer be able to promote themselves as waterproof since no product is completely waterproof, nor can it be marketed as "sun block" since nothing can completely block the sun's rays. Labels must now use words like "water resistant," and they must state how long, in minutes, the product will resist water before it must be reapplied.

The newer guidelines are meant to help consumers avoid confusion about which sun care products actually protect them from cancer and premature aging. A sun product that provides broad spectrum protection against both UVA and UVB rays with an SPF of 15 or higher *can* state that it will protect against cancer and premature aging. If a sunscreen is not a broad spectrum protectant (e.g., only protects against UVA **OR** UVB rays—not both), it cannot state that it will help prevent cancer or skin aging.

## Steps to Take to Deter Wrinkles

Many people have occupations that keep them outdoors all the time—farmers and fisherman for example—and they are constantly exposed to the sun.

Recreational activities like swimming, sailing, and other outdoor sports like golfing, tennis, baseball, and soccer expose participants to the sun and the weather. It is therefore essential that people participating in these types of activities be well protected.

An adequate broad spectrum sunscreen is essential for anyone that spends a lot of time outdoors, particularly those with sensitive or fair skin that is more prone to sunburn. An SPF of 15 or more provides good protection against the sun's harmful UVA and UVB rays.

Clothing plays a major part in protecting the skin and minimizing the risks of exposure to the sun. Wearing a hat protects the top of the head, which is especially vulnerable if you have short or thin hair. A hat with a wide brim protects the face as well. Long sleeves cover the arms and pants or long dresses limit exposure to the legs. All of these precautions help deter wrinkles and fine lines.

## ❖ How to Choose the Right Skin Product for You

Skincare is a very competitive business and consumers are inundated with information about hundreds of skincare products for every possible skin type, so how do you choose the best skincare products for you? How do you know what skin type you have? Here are a few tips for making smart and educated choices for a healthy skincare regime.

❖ Identify your skin type. This is not rocket science, and you don't need a consultant or physician to type your skin; what you need is a mirror and some good old fashioned honesty. Using a large mirror, take a close look at your clean face. Be sure to position yourself where the lighting is natural and bright. Examine your face for dry areas; note the size of your pores—are there any skin rashes or acne present; do you have any black heads, white heads, open lesions, or dark areas; and what is the color tone like?

❖ Determine if your skin is mostly dry, mostly oily, or a combination of both. You are the best judge of how your skin feels and reacts to your daily routine. You know if your skin is oily in the heat of summer and dry during the cold, harsh winter. Maybe your skin is only oily around the nose and forehead. Blot your clean, dry face with a tissue and then look at the tissue to see if there are any oily spots. Make notes on your observations about your skin before you shop for skincare products.

## What to look for in a skincare product

When you decide to start a new skincare routine, it is always a good idea to shop around for products that best suit your skin type. Most consumers choose products with four main ideas in mind. These are:

❖ Cost

❖ Scent and Feel

❖ Purpose

❖ Expected Results

## Choosing Products

Regardless of where you shop, choose products made for your specific skin type. If you have oily skin, choose oil-free products. Conversely, if you have dry skin, choose a product made specifically for that skin type—one that contains extra moisturizing ingredients to keep the skin from becoming excessively dry. Products for skin that is both oily *and* dry are called combination skincare products and are made to address both the dry and the oily areas of your skin.

Look for products with natural ingredients like vitamins and minerals; avoid products with harsh chemicals and alcohols which may cause skin irritation or allergic reactions for some skin types.

## Price Points to Consider

❖ Choose products in a price range you can easily afford.

❖ Read labels and compare ingredients, quality, scent, and price.

❖ Shop online for the product or an equivalent skincare product to realize additional savings.

It may take a recommendation from a friend, some research, or just some plain old trial and error before you find the right products for you.

## Tips to Consider for Your Safety

❖ Most products made by the same company are designed to work together. You may find greater satisfaction and better results when you purchase the skincare products from the same line.

❖ When searching for the right products for your skin type, introduce only one new product or line at a time. If you develop an allergic reaction or skin irritation, it will be easier to discover which product caused the symptoms.

❖ Use the products that feel best to you. Products your friends suggest may feel great to them, but they may make your skin feel dry and itchy. The product is only as good as it makes you look and feel, regardless of what the marketing hype claims.

The main considerations in the selection of good skincare products are how they make you look, how they feel on your skin, and how comfortable you are with the performance and pricing of the products. When you find products that work with your skin type, stay with them for a younger, healthier look and feel.

## How to Choose a Good Anti-Wrinkle Product

Maintaining a youthful appearance is probably the single most important factor people consider when buying cosmetics. With so many anti-aging skin products available in stores and online, selecting the right protection can seem like a daunting task. So how do we choose the right and, more importantly, the most effective age-defying products?

## Choose a Product for Your Skin Type

Not all skin types are alike. Each has a specific set of needs that must be met in order to provide effective anti-aging protection. No single cream will be suitable for every user. If your skin is dry or mature, a heavier, moisture-rich, anti-wrinkle product is the most suitable for you. If you have normal, combination, or oily skin, a moisture serum or gel will be more effective.

## Familiarize Yourself with Key Ingredients

With such a wide variety of anti-wrinkle products being advertised, many of us have become quite familiar with the names of key ingredients, but we actually have no idea what each ingredient does. For instance, you may be very familiar with terms like retinol, lanolin, polyphenols, and coenzyme Q10, yet wonder what they can do for your skin — are they right for your skin type? Before buying, take the time to do some research on the effectiveness of the ingredients contained in anti-aging skincare products.

## Consider the following prior to purchase

❖ Do the ingredients stimulate skin regeneration or renewal?

❖ Are they present in levels that will actually be effective?

❖ Do any of the inactive ingredients interfere with the effectiveness of the active ingredients?

❖ Which technology is used to deliver the ingredients into skin?

❖ Are any ingredients potentially harmful to skin?

A little research and forethought will make you less susceptible to the latest industry gimmicks and help you make informed decisions about the anti-aging skincare that is best suited to your needs.

Another important consideration when you look at ingredients is the levels of concentration. The concentration is a major factor in the effectiveness of an anti wrinkle cream. Some products have the right ingredients as part of their formulas, but they are not in the concentrations recommended in studies, and the product will therefore not be effective.

The following ingredients should always meet these minimum concentrations:

❖ 1% Sodium Hyaluronate

❖ 3% Matrixyl 3000

❖ 10% Argireline

# Learn About the Technology Behind The Cream

Similar to our lack of knowledge about common anti-aging ingredients, most consumers usually have very little understanding of the technology behind the cosmetics they purchase. Cosmetic companies are aware of this and use it to their advantage. In order not to be misled by these modern-day snake oil salesmen, it is vital that you research and understand the technologies that support ingredient delivery.

## Consider the Reputation of the Company

Companies spend billions each year to ensure their reputations remain unsullied in the public eye. According to their websites and television commercials, the companies advertizing the products are the most effective and offer the best value on the market. In order to really put a company's reputation to the test, consumers need to look for unbiased, completely objective reviews of the company and its products. While cosmetics salespeople may seem very knowledgeable about products they sell, they are not unbiased, and often they aren't even experts about the products.

To find objective opinions, consult friends, family, coworkers, and acquaintances. The Internet is another valuable source of information. Consumer-oriented websites and forums provide a wealth of information on the standing of a company and the effectiveness of the products they sell.

## ❖ Does Anti-Wrinkle Cream Actually Work?

Every day, consumers are inundated with marketing that targets one of our greatest fears: aging. Cosmetic companies promise to make us look younger through regular application of their new, age-defying creams that are packed full of active compounds taken from exotic plant extracts. By playing on our fear of growing old, using slogans with scientific sounding terms or rare sounding ingredients, and throwing around the word 'research', these companies lead us to believe that youth is really available in a jar. But how can a person be sure these products are really effective in preventing or reversing the aging process?

Consider the following points before buying into industry promises.

### The Bitter Truth

Most of the claims and promises made about products in the cosmetic industry are untrue. Nearly 80% of the anti-aging products on the market do not live up to the claims made about them. That means only one product in five will actually produce the results advertised. The only way to be sure you are using an effective anti-aging product is to do your homework. Look for product comparisons done by unbiased consumer testing organizations and read online consumer forums that offer feedback from actual consumers, not paid bloggers.

### Do Some Research of Your Own

One of the most effective sales gimmicks cosmetic companies use to market their anti-aging products is the use of words and phrases geared to trigger scientific credibility in our minds. Through the use of expressions like, "six out of ten users say...," "Clinical research shows...," or "Laboratory tests conclude that...," we are led to believe their promises and end up paying huge sums of money for glorified moisturizing products.

Before you buy anything, check the company's clinical evidence. Find out if the research was done by the company's own laboratory (which is often the case) or if the research was actually done by a scientifically or academically reputable testing institution.

## Get Ingredient Smart

Another marketing ploy used to plug anti-aging products is the use of terms like "extracts," "essences" and "infusions," all purported to be from exotic-sounding plants, herbs, or berries. This may make the product sound more exclusive and luxurious, but beware. The effectiveness of these ingredients is doubtful. Before deciding on an anti-wrinkle cream, look up its active ingredients. Is there any unbiased clinical research to suggest it really works? Examine the other ingredients. Do they interact with each other in a negative way by reducing shelf life or perhaps counteracting the effects of the active ingredients? And, most importantly, are any of the ingredients known to be harmful? Armed with this knowledge, you will be less likely to succumb to clever advertising traps.

## ❖ FIVE LIFESTYLE MISTAKES THAT LEAD TO WRINKLES

The old adage about *an ounce of prevention* could have been written about those pesky fine lines and wrinkles that begin to make their appearance much sooner than we might have liked. Slowing the aging process is often just a matter of making simple lifestyle changes that effectively protect the skin and keep it looking younger for a much longer time.

Avoid these five lifestyle mistakes that can lead to the appearance of wrinkles, and then implement the simple changes suggested here to begin your preventative, anti-aging regimen today.

## Mistake #1: Choosing other Beverages over Water

Failing to give your body the hydration it needs can lead to sagging skin and wrinkles. There is no easier anti-aging program than making sure you consume at least eight glasses of water every day. Feel free to add an occasional glass of red wine or a daily cup of green tea to your beverage program as well, since their high levels of antioxidants protect the skin from free radical damage and act as natural anti-aging elements.

## Mistake #2: Sleeping in Your Makeup

Leaving makeup on overnight clogs pores and prevents your skin from getting much needed time to breathe and recover from the stresses of the day. Remove makeup daily with a cleanser that is appropriate for your skin type and follow up with a moisturizer that keeps your skin soft and supple.

## Mistake #3: Postponing the Use of Skincare Products

You are never too young to begin an anti-aging skincare regimen that keeps free radicals at bay and promotes collagen and elastin production in the skin.

Begin your anti-aging regimen as early as possible. It is much easier to prevent fine lines than it is to mask deeper wrinkles once they arrive. For best results, find products suitable to your age and skin type and get your regimen underway.

## Mistake #4: Allowing Stress to Reign

Stress is a natural byproduct of our busy lives, but that doesn't mean we have to allow stress to take its toll on our skin. Find ways to manage stress through exercise, meditation, and other activities. Get a good night's sleep every night to give the body time to recharge and rejuvenate. Avoid stressed-out people who only serve to raise your blood pressure without providing constructive benefit to your life.

## Mistake #5: Eating High Fat, Sugary Foods

Your skin is the largest organ of your body, and it makes sense that the foods you put into your body affect your skin. Skin looks best when it is fed a diet rich in nutrients like antioxidants and omega-3 fatty acids. Avoid pore-clogging fare like fried foods and those high in sugar to make your skin look more radiant and youthful from the inside out.

There is no doubt that many women worry about the effects of aging their skin, as evidenced by the number of anti-aging products on the market today. Keeping skin looking younger is often a matter of changing simple lifestyle habits. By avoiding these five common mistakes, you can enjoy younger, more radiant-looking skin throughout your life.

## ◈ FIVE STEPS TO PREVENT WRINKLES

While wrinkles may be inevitable, there are ways to prevent the development of additional lines and crow's feet, as well as ways to conceal those that already exist.

**Keep exposure to the sun to a minimum.** What many people perceive as signs of aging are actually signs of sun damage. Try to avoid the sun from 10 a.m. to 4 p.m., when the sun is at its hottest. When you do go out, wear sunscreen, a hat, sunglasses, cotton blend clothing, and shirts with long sleeves.

**Always wear sunscreen.** According to Dr. Sandra I. Read, an instructor of dermatology at the Georgetown University School of Medicine, you should apply sunscreen with a sun protection factor (SPF) of at least 15 or 30. It is important to use a sunscreen that offers broad-spectrum protection from both types of damaging rays.

**Never downplay the importance of a healthy diet.** The foods you eat make a profound difference in your body—both inside and out. Eat a diet rich in fruits and vegetables, whole grains, lean meats, and seafood. In addition, supplement your diet with plenty of vitamins, minerals and antioxidants to improve the overall appearance of your skin.

**If you smoke, stop.** If you don't smoke, don't start. Smoking is bad for the skin and brings about premature wrinkling. The skin around the mouth is particularly susceptible to wrinkling, dryness, and a dull appearance due to smoking.

**Use a good moisturizer** for your skin, and use it faithfully. Dr. Brandt, Strivectin, and Murad are all excellent moisturizers to try. Use different moisturizers for the daytime and the nighttime. Daytime moisturizers should be light weight and water-based. They should be applied after washing your face in the morning in order to lock moisture into your skin.

Choose a daytime moisturizer that contains SPF. For nighttime, choose a moisturizer that is heavier and that protects and moisturizes your skin while you are sleeping. Be aware that changing seasons and temperatures can affect the condition of your skin, and that you will have to change your moisturizer accordingly. In terms of anti-aging skincare, look for moisturizers that contain glycolic acid, retinol, peptides, Sodium Hyaluronate, matrixyl 3000 and Syn-coll.

These ingredients promote the growth of collagen, which combats wrinkles and counteracts free radicals.

**Note:** AHAs, a common ingredient in anti-aging products, can be irritating to the skin, so test the product on a small patch of skin before applying it all over your face.

## ◈ 5 BEAUTY TIPS FOR PROTECTING YOURSELF FROM THE SUN

We all love spending time in the sun, whether we're soaking up deliciously warm rays on the beach or enjoying a bright afternoon on the front porch. However, sun exposure can damage the skin, accelerate the aging process and may even contribute to the risk of some types of cancer. With that in mind, we need to take steps to protect ourselves from excessive sun exposure, and there are plenty of ways to do so.

**Minimize exposure** — The main way to protect your skin is to minimize your exposure to the sun. During the summer, between the hours of 10 a.m. and 2 p.m., the body is much more susceptible to damaging rays. If possible, stay out of the sun during this peak time. If you must work in the sun, apply adequate sun protection.

**Watch the clouds** — Year-round protection is essential to a good skincare regimen. Sun protection is still necessary during the winter months since snow and ice reflect the sun's rays. On cloudy days, the sun can be extremely dangerous as it penetrates the clouds without people realizing it.

**Know your vulnerabilities** — Some medications and skincare products make you more vulnerable to the damaging effects of the sun. Ask your doctor if the medications he is prescribing for you can make your skin more likely to burn. Look at the label on your skincare products to see if there is a warning about sun exposure. If so, be extra vigilant about protection, consistently applying sunscreen daily before leaving your house.

**Best sun protection** — There are many sunscreen products to choose from, but some brands offer better protection than others. Look for a product with a high SPF, particularly if you have fair skin. Yonka offers a sunscreen with an SPF 40 specifically designed for those with skin more vulnerable to the sun's rays. It is also important to inspect the ingredients used to provide protection. One of the best is zinc oxide, a key ingredient in Fenix sun care products. Both Yonka and Fenix products slow the effects of aging and reduce the risk of skin cancer due to sun exposure.

People with oily skin often dislike using sunscreen because it clogs pores and leads to breakouts. G.M. Collin offers a sunscreen specifically for oily skin. It offers adequate protection from the sun without contributing to breakouts. G.M. Collin also offers a comprehensive line of other sun protection products designed for every need and skin type.

**UV filters and SPF levels** — Anthelios SX from La Roche Posay is an SPF 15 moisturizer that protects the skin from UVA and UVB rays through an ingredient called Mexoryl SX that acts as a UV filter. It protects skin cells and helps you maintain a youthful appearance. Applying this sun protection to the face daily not only filters UV rays but also keeps the skin hydrated.

Peter Thomas Roth's oil-free sun block is another product that effectively protects skin to ward off aging. It is a powerful SPF 30 product that is fragrance-free and non-irritating and can be used on all skin types. Using a sun block, whether at the beach or in the mountains skiing, is advisable as sea water, sand, and snow are very reflective and can increase the sun's damaging rays by up to 80%.

Using sun protection as a regular part of your skincare routine is just common sense — protect your skin from the elements and maintain your skin's vitality. Sun protection keeps your skin looking youthful, vibrant, and hydrated.

## ◈ Moisturizers 101: Choosing the Right One

One of the most important steps in a daily beauty regimen is moisturizer. However, many people don't think they need moisturizer unless they have noticeably dry skin. Usually, this is not the case. The skin loses moisture at almost every turn.

Cosmetics can rob the skin of vital oils, and even soaps and cleansers can strip away the skin's natural moisture balance. Free radicals, harsh weather conditions, and the sun deplete the skin's natural hydration even further, and aging can be caused by dehydration. A daily application of an oil-free moisturizer is critical to maintain the skin's proper balance and prevent many adverse skin conditions.

Moisturizers come in many forms, but the main thing consumers should keep in mind is that moisturizers should be oil-free. Products that contain oil clog the pores and lead to unsightly blemishes, blackheads, and whiteheads. Skincare companies have spent years developing moisturizers in the form of gels, lotions, creams, mists, and serums. The specific type chosen depends primarily on individual preference—some creams may be too heavy for sensitive skin, while mists may not provide enough moisturizer for extremely dry skin.

Consumers that want more than just hydration from their moisturizers should choose a product with dual or triple functions. Many moisturizers contain an SPF for added protection from the sun, while some also include ingredients to fight blemishes or brighten the skin. A tinted moisturizer provides subtle coverage in place of a foundation. Those individuals that use a daily moisturizer frequently find the aging process is slowed and rough patches are avoided.

## Choosing a Moisturizer

When shopping for a moisturizer, consider these factors:

❖ Skin type (dry, oily, normal, combination)

❖ Specific needs (acne treatment, anti-aging, etc.)

❖ The big picture for your full regimen (if you need sun protection, you need to find a moisturizer with an SPF)

❖ The ingredients (avoid fragrances and artificial dyes that can irritate sensitive skin)

You may find that the product that works best on your face isn't as effective on the delicate eye area or on rougher spots like the elbows. Many women choose a different moisturizer for each of these areas in order to get the optimum results from their products, so the best moisturizer for you may actually turn out to be a combination of several products.

## ◈ Using a Moisturizer

Apply moisturizer to damp skin whenever possible. This allows the product to lock in extra moisture and hydrate the skin for a longer period of time. Very dry areas, such as the hands and feet, may benefit from a rich slathering of moisturizer while the skin is still damp. Swaddle them in a pair of cotton socks or gloves to help the moisturizer absorb into the skin more effectively.

### Clayton Shagal

One brand of moisturizer to consider is Clayton Shagal. This company understands the importance of hydration, which is why they combine deep and surface moisturizing ingredients to create the most thorough treatment possible. The Clayton Shagal moisturizing products are appropriate for any skin type—some work specifically to minimize skin breakouts or treat aging skin.

### Ageless Derma Stem Cell and Peptide Anti-wrinkle Cream

This product protects the skin from the signs of aging using seven natural, anti-aging ingredients. Ageless Derma Stem Cell and Peptide Anti-Wrinkle Cream eliminates fine lines and wrinkles, improves firmness and elasticity, eliminates crow's feet, and re-energizes skin.

### DDF Skincare

DDF understands that hydrated skin is firmer and younger-looking, so the products in its line are designed to heal and protect while adding necessary moisture. Advanced Firming Cream is one of the top products for this purpose; in addition to providing important moisturizing ingredients like shea butter, this formula also contains peptides to boost the skin's own collagen production and a turmeric complex to protect the skin from further damage.

## Dermalogica

Dermalogica provides a wide line of moisturizers to address every need and skin type. The collection offers a tinted moisturizer to wear in place of foundation and a number of products with SPF to protect the skin as they hydrate. For people with aging skin, the Dermalogica Power Rich System offers hydrating ingredients designed to increase collagen production and firm skin. These products do not contain artificial fragrances or colors, so they are safe for even the most sensitive skin types.

Moisturizer is an important step in any skincare regimen. The right moisturizer hydrates the skin, leaving it softer, smoother and younger-looking.

## ◈ How to Look Younger with Anti-Aging Mineral Makeup

It seems that every Hollywood diva, from Madonna to Julia Roberts, has hopped aboard the mineral makeup bandwagon. The popularity of these all-natural cosmetics has prompted real-life beauty gurus to take notice. Why are celebrities and professional makeup artists so enthusiastic about foundation and blush created from finely ground minerals? We're going to discuss why you might want to try the latest mineral makeup and offer you some tips to help you find the best formulas for your skin.

Mineral makeup has been used for centuries, but recently it has enjoyed a resurgence of popularity. Mineral makeup has been touted as better for the skin because the all-natural formulas are devoid of artificial fragrances, dyes, and preservatives. However, the benefits may go well beyond the "natural" moniker.

## Benefits of Mineral Makeup

Here are several reasons to consider mineral makeup for a cleaner, healthier complexion. Mineral makeup:

❖ Provides much lighter coverage by using a unique blend of chemical-free, all-natural ingredients

❖ Feels lighter without adversely affecting coverage— flaws like scars and fine lines seem to disappear

❖ Won't damage the skin's surface

❖ Lasts longer than other types of makeup

❖ Offers better coverage for a flawless complexion

❖ Reduces the risk of breakouts since pores aren't clogged

❖ Won't irritate the skin

In addition to these benefits, some women find that mineral makeup can even turn back the clock.

## How Mineral Makeup Fights Aging Skin

One of the primary causes of aging skin is the sun. Sunlight leads to dry, sagging skin and the appearance of fine lines and wrinkles. It is important to protect your skin, but you don't need thick sunscreens that could produce breakouts or irritation. Mineral makeup offers a hefty dose of sun-protecting agents like zinc oxide and titanium dioxide in their formulas. Some mineral makeup products provide SPFs as high as 30 to protect the delicate skin of your face.

One ingredient to **avoid** in mineral makeup is bismuth oxychloride. This substance is frequently used in mineral formulas to enhance the glow of the skin, but bismuth oxychloride has also been shown to irritate skin, and it can make some existing skin conditions worse. If you have sensitive skin or a chronic skin condition, avoid mineral makeup that lists this ingredient.

## Recommended Mineral Makeup Lines

Not all mineral makeup companies are created equal. It is important to look for companies that use only natural ingredients, void of artificial dyes, perfumes, or preservatives. Choose mineral makeup that has added vitamins, antioxidants, and green tea extract for better skin care.

**Jane Iredale** is one such company that is recommended by dermatologists and cosmetic surgeons because it is safe and offers many benefits. The state-of-the-art formulas created by Jane Iredale come in a wide range of shades to suit every skin tone.

**Colorescience** is another good mineral makeup source. This company uses only the highest quality ingredients in their formulas. These products are packed with important nutrients like antioxidants and enzymes that treat the skin even as they provide a more beautiful complexion.

**Ageless Derma Mineral Makeup** is healthy for your skin and made in the United States. It is made of all natural, top quality ingredients that offer flawless coverage and flattering colors for all skin types. The products are strong enough to protect the skin from harsh UVA and UVB rays, yet they nourish the skin and are gentle enough to use immediately after cosmetic surgery.

**Glominerals** offers a wide line of cosmetics in fashion-forward shades with a few color classics included for good measure.

## ◈ MARVELOUS TIPS ON HOW FOOD AFFECTS YOUR SKIN

Soft, smooth, creamy skin is what we all crave, but very often—particularly as we age—our skin loses its youthful bloom. Our skin needs nourishment and care just as our bodies do, and if we mistreat our skin it very often ages prematurely and becomes dull and dry. So what can be done?

Start with the foods that you eat every day. They can have a huge impact on how your skin looks and feels. That doesn't mean you have to eat exotic foods, spend a fortune on treatments, or slave over a stove all day—quite the opposite. Eating right is actually quite simple and will go a long way toward improving your skin and restoring its natural beauty.

**Water**—It is amazing how much water can do for your skin. It's a well-known fact that you are supposed to drink eight glasses of water every day, but how many of us actually do that? People that get plenty of water enjoy skin that is more hydrated and nourished. Water is a natural cleanser for the body; it flushes out toxins and makes an observable difference in the complexion.

**Avocado**—Contains niacin, an anti-inflammatory that keeps the skin soothed and calm. This fruit nourishes the skin with essential oils and B-complex vitamins. It can be used as a mask to replenish dry skin.

**Cottage cheese**—This dairy product has calcium, in itself good for you, and selenium, an essential mineral that combats free radicals. It will also protect the skin against cancer.

**Mushrooms** — People with rosacea or sensitive skin prone to blemishes can benefit from mushrooms. Loaded with riboflavin, mushrooms are reparative, and an excellent menu addition for people who have had surgery or suffered a wound. Mushrooms promote balance in the skin.

**Baked potato** (with the skin left on to take advantage of full benefits) — Enriched with copper, potatoes help the skin heal. They also work with other essential minerals to restore the skin's elasticity and support structure.

**Berries and cherries** — Many berries (e.g., blueberries, blackberries, black grapes, black currants, acai berries, and cherries) are rich in antioxidants that protect the skin against free radical damage

**Orange fruits and vegetables** — Foods like mangoes and carrots are rich in Vitamin A which repairs the skin and fights free radical damage. They are low in calories, making them ideal for dieters.

**Almonds and nuts** — These contain huge amounts of vitamin E. Almonds are rich in essential oils that nourish the skin and keep it moisturized, and they contain antioxidants to fight free radicals. Walnuts and other nuts provide protein — essential to collagen production which translates to better elasticity.

These are just some of the foods that can enhance your skin's appearance, keep it in better repair and constantly replenish it. Ingesting large quantities of antioxidants (found in berries and foods like pomegranate, ginger, and sunflower seeds) protect the skin and fight free radical damage so the skin is better conditioned and more radiant.

Proteins found in meats, nuts, beans, and other foods are important to the skin. They keep the skin's collagen production active and enhance elasticity. The Omega-3 fatty acids found in flaxseed oil and walnuts are important to keep skin cells strong. They allow the skin to retain water, making it smooth and soft.

## ◈ SKINCARE TABLETS FOR BEAUTIFUL SKIN

Beauty is not only external. Our skin and our faces are just the wrapper for the inner aspects of our physical well-being. We can actually enhance the appearance of our skin by taking skincare tablets, which are loaded with valuable nutrients.

Aging is an inevitable, natural process. Products have been formulated that include natural anti-aging elements. VitaMedica has developed a line of products based on this premise, including VitaMedica Arnica Montana, which is used in the recovery stage of post-operative cosmetic procedures.

Many people, especially women, are very conscious of the appearance of their skin and worry about whether or not they have visible cellulite. They spend thousands of dollars annually on products targeting such issues, but their efforts will be worthless if they don't look for products that provide what the body needs. To address this condition, the Murad Company developed The Murad Firm and Tone Dietary Supplement.

In addition to skincare tablets, Borba introduced a powder mix taken orally that contains vital nutrients and antioxidants. It is especially effective against wrinkles, discoloration, and other tell-tale signs of aging.

## ◈ THE HARMFUL EFFECTS OF STRESS ON THE SKIN

German scientists at the University of Dresden found that a particular stress hormone interacts with a receptor in the skin and causes damaging inflammation that results in wrinkles. Stress has a huge impact on the way we feel and act, but many people do not realize that it also has a harmful effect on the skin. Stress wreaks havoc both inside and outside of our bodies.

## Exacerbates Other Conditions

Stress or anxiety can cause any condition in the body to worsen. For people with acne or sensitive skin prone to blemishes, stress can cause the outbreak of lesions. Those with excessive perspiration or hair loss may see their problems increase, and those with psoriasis or rosacea may find that their skin is more inflamed and redder than usual. Stress can cause the skin to become dehydrated which, in turn, allows all types of infectious allergens to penetrate the skin. Conditions like eczema and rashes can occur and breakouts may be more frequent.

People under a lot of stress may become depressed and neglect daily skincare. Their skin could well become itchy and dry starting a vicious cycle of scratching, rubbing, and increased irritation. Neglect can cause a breakdown in the normal repair and restoration cycle the skin goes through as it rids itself of dead cells. Skin that is dehydrated cannot recover if left untreated.

## Effects on Your Skin

Stress can cause fever blisters, dermatitis and other skin conditions that you might not normally develop. Your nails may turn brittle and you may break out in hives. Long-term stress can cause intensely adverse effects on the skin such as poor circulation, and the decreased blood supply to the skin can make it flaky, dry, and irritated. Stress can affect your respiratory system, reducing the amount of oxygen supplied to the skin. This causes the skin to appear dull and pasty and to lose its natural glow.

If your skin is lacking all the things that are important to keep it healthy—blood, oxygen and water—it becomes dull and gray. People with nutrient-deprived skin develop puffiness and dark circles around the eyes, and wrinkles and fine lines may increase and deepen.

## Stress Seeks Comfort

When we are under stress, we tend to eat and drink the wrong things, like coffee or alcohol that are debilitating, dehydrating, and drying to the skin. This is the time when you should be increasing your water intake to keep the skin moisturized and nourished, but because of anxiety and depression, you reach for things that are harmful instead. The next time you're feeling stressed, reach for the fruits and vegetables and forget the *comfort foods* that don't nourish the body or the skin. Giving in to impulse eating and drinking is a downward spiral that is difficult to escape. It is important to seek help if you feel like stress is gaining control in your life. Long-term stress can cause irreparable damage if left untreated, but the good news is that it can be diagnosed and treated by a qualified physician.

## Coping With Stress

It's easy to say that you should reduce stress, but it's one of those things that is often easier to talk about than to do. Making some time for yourself, just an hour each day, to perform some of the skincare rituals mentioned in this book can help reduce the effects of stress on your skin, and it can help you mentally too. Exercise and relaxation techniques work wonders. Once you start seeing the effects of wrinkle creams or other skincare treatments, you will inevitably notice that you have a more hopeful outlook too. You start to feel stronger and are better able to cope with stress when you look and feel your best.

## ◈ Beautiful Skin, Beautiful Body: Why Skincare is Not Just for Your Face

Skin is the largest organ of the body, yet many people focus their skincare regimen on the face alone. While it is important to treat your complexion right, you shouldn't ignore the rest of your body in the process. Some of the most challenging skin issues can occur in other parts of the body such as the elbows, heels, and shoulders. By caring for all of your skin, you put more than your best face forward everyday; you'll flaunt a beautiful body as well.

## Skincare for the Body

Most skincare products are designed specifically for either the face or the body. The face has different needs than the rest of your skin. For example, a rich, hydrating formula that smoothes rough patches on the feet will clog pores and result in breakouts if used on the face. By the same token, ingredients used to tighten skin and stimulate collagen production on the face won't provide do much for your legs and arms. Do yourself a favor and choose one set of skincare products for your face and another for the rest of your body.

## What to Look for in Body Skincare

Skincare products for the body should serve a dual purpose—hydrating dry skin and protecting it from further damage. A moisturizer with an SPF offers both benefits in a single formula that is both convenient and good value. Body skincare can also offer other advantages, such as minimizing the effects of cellulite, reducing stretch marks, and tightening flabby skin on problem areas like the stomach and buttocks. As with facial skincare products, look for those that address your specific needs and skin type.

## PCA Skin

PCA Skin is one of the few skincare companies that offer products that can be used on both the face and body. Perfecting Face and Body Hydrator is a formula rich in sun protection, and it treats a host of skin imperfections. PCA Skin is a leading company in the development of both professional and home skincare products. It specializes in peels and advanced topical solutions that address a wide cross-section of needs.

## La Roche Posay

La Roche Posay provides some excellent hydrating formulas for the skin. Their Lipikar Body Balm is particularly effective on problem areas where dry, flaky skin can develop. The product is potent enough that a single application each day is enough to produce the desired results. A great side benefit is that it doesn't leave oily or greasy residue on the skin. This moisturizer is excellent when used in combination with Lipikar Bath Oil and offers extra moisturizing benefits.

## Rodial

Rodial offers one of the best lines in body care, with formulas that do everything from tightening the tummy to erasing stretch marks. Most of the body care products target specific areas, although a few, like Powder Body Buff and Crème de la Crème, are designed to work on the whole body. Rodial products contain high quality ingredients that sculpt and tone the body through topical solutions.

When planning a skincare regimen, don't leave your body out in the cold. With a complete skincare program, you'll be putting your best foot, face, and body forward every day.

## ❖ ANTI-AGING SKINCARE GUIDE FOR MEN

While the bulk of the anti-aging products on the market are directed at women, there are a significant number of men who also want to turn back the clock. However, the delicate fragrances and pretty packaging typical in women's products aren't the best choices for a man's skin.

Thankfully, many top skincare companies have lines of anti-aging skincare created specifically for men. In the next section, we'll explore the basics of men's anti-aging skincare and provide a few recommendations that can help even the most macho guys slow the aging process.

## Why Men's Skin Ages Differently from Women's

Although men and women go through a similar aging process, the symptoms of aging differ between the genders. While women lose collagen, men face a serious deficit in hydration that can lead to the appearance of fine lines and sagging skin. Anti-aging products for men are most often focused on restoring that hydration rather than on promoting collagen production. This explains why ingredients like peptides are often absent from men's anti-aging products, while hydrating ingredients like sodium hyaluronate are a definite must.

Men tend to be harder on their skin than women; they spend more time in the sun and subject their faces to the daily irritation of shaving. It is important to find anti-aging products that combat the effects of sun damage through the addition of antioxidants that also help to repair the skin. Shaving irritation is a problem, so moisturizing ingredients that soothe rough skin are also important in a man's anti-aging regimen. There are two companies that provide men's anti-aging lines that address these male-specific issues.

**Yonka** — Yonka is a broad skincare line for both men and women, with a variety of products designed just for their male clientele. Yonka Age Defense provides a blend of active ingredients that promise to increase hydrations by 115% just two hours after applying, and it contains antioxidants that protect the skin from further damage. This Yonka product can be used effectively after the effects of aging have already set in, but if you start your program early, you can stop the damage before it starts.

**Babor** — Babor skincare for men includes two products specifically geared to address the effects of aging. Babor's Energizing Age Preventing Cream offers a variety of proteins to minimize the appearance of fine lines and wrinkles, while panthenol and bisabolol provide the hydration a man's skin needs. Babor's Line Reducing Eye Gel directs its action at one of the prime problem spots for men — the fine lines and crow's feet that appear around the eyes.

Anti-aging is not just a concern for women. With skincare lines designed just for the male population, men can also enjoy smoother, younger looking skin.

# ಬಿ 2 ಛ

# ANTI-AGING SKINCARE FOR THE EYES, EYELASHES AND LIPS

## ◈ EYES AND EYELASHES

## Say Good Bye to Puffy Eyes and Dark Circles for Good

T he eyes are often referred to as the windows to the soul. They are also among man's most noticeable features. They must be well cared for as our skin is constantly exposed to damaging, toxic elements, and the skin around the eyes is the thinnest and most delicate tissue on the body. Puffy eyes occur due to things like excessive crying and allergies. Crying causes the eyes to redden and swell, resulting in eye irritation.

Hormonal changes, stress, alcohol, and lack of sleep are also detrimental to the tissue around the eyes. Another problem, unsightly dark circles, is usually the result of lack of sleep, nasal congestion, and/or vitamin deficiency. The most alarming aspect of puffy eyes for beauty-conscious people is that it can lead to premature aging that manifests through the emergence of wrinkles, lines, and crow's feet. Fortunately, there are now many good anti-aging skincare products to counteract these visual assaults on our faces, necks, and hands; specifically, there are now eye creams that effectively combat the signs of aging and diminish dark circles and puffiness around the eyes. A good eye cream is a beauty necessity.

## Conventional Versus Contemporary Eye Treatment

Two widely used home remedies for fighting puffiness and dark circles are cucumbers and green tea bags. Though traditionally believed to reduce the swelling and remove unwanted shadows around the eyes, the fact is that they only provide short-term relief through their cooling effect on the skin. Similarly, applying eye makeup is a short-term solution as it only covers up the existing problem.

Modern science is constantly developing new anti-aging skincare that can have lasting effects on the eyes, and the purchase of an eye cream that has been scientifically formulated to eliminate puffiness and dark circles is surely a wise investment. Ageless Derma Eye Cream is a powerful new anti-aging treatment that helps to prevent and reverse the signs of aging. Its unique formula combines Retinol, the purest form of Vitamin A, with Vitamins C, E and K to soften the appearance of dark circles, smooth fine lines and wrinkles and improve skin texture around the delicate eye area

Another product worth mentioning is Vivier's Dark Circle Diminishing Eye Cream. It contains a valuable mixture of vitamins C and K. Vitamin C is a powerful antioxidant, while vitamin K has restorative properties. Massaging this product into the eye area daily has provided noticeable results.

## Free Yourself from Worn Out Eyes

Few things are more beautiful and more representative of good health than a young woman's eyes. However, things like work, outdoor recreation, and busy schedules can make eyes look tired—dark circles may appear and premature aging may also set in. Hylexin is a product that helps prevent capillaries from leaking by providing a good atmosphere for enzymatic processes to occur. Bremenn Research Labs manufactures Hylexin and its clients have had a 72% success rate in lightening dark circles. Hylexin can be used on sensitive parts of the eye because it is non-comedogenic, hypoallergenic, and scent-free.

Ageless Derma Eye Cream is an effective product for dark circles around the eyes. It contains powerful antioxidants, coenzyme 10, Sodium Hyaluronate, vitamins A, K, E and C, Retinol, Argireline and peptides. Research done in the Department of Dermatology, Nippon Medical School, Tokyo, Japan, indicates that this combination of ingredients is very effective in eliminating dark circle around the eyes.

## Products that Reduce Eye Puffiness

Your skin type and lifestyle are unique to you, and as you age, it's important to understand how to choose the best eye care products to complement your needs. Factors like age, the level of repair and restoration needed, the amount of hydration needed, and the nutritional requirements for your skin should all play a role in your skincare purchasing decisions. Anti-aging products, particularly those products that treat puffiness around the eyes, are always evolving and becoming more sophisticated. With so many products on the market, choosing a good eye treatment can be difficult.

Our experts have done the research and know — both from scientific study and through consumer feedback — which anti-aging skincare products contain the most effective blends of ingredients to reduce the appearance of puffiness around the eyes. We believe the products discussed in this book are among the best skincare products currently on the market. However, we are constantly researching new products and reevaluating our choices.

## Gorgeous Eyelashes Celebrities Would Envy

Only a select few are born with naturally long and voluptuous eyelashes. The movie stars who don't have them create them. Celebrities are often asked to endorse beauty products like mascara in television commercials and print ads. Celebrities are not necessarily naturally beautiful; they often need help to look their best, and you can look your best too by getting in touch with the latest breakthrough products in the cosmetics industry.

Most people don't think to include eyelash treatment as part of their beauty regimen. However, eyelashes are incredibly sensitive to harsh chemicals and should be treated with special care. Many consumers suffer from thinning eyelashes, and sometimes their eyelashes are simply too short. In order to promote eyelash growth and health, a proper eyelash treatment should be used regularly. There are many companies that supply eyelash treatments, but people should only purchase those with a longstanding reputation in the cosmetic industry.

Talika is a cosmetics company that emerged from a surprising discovery. In 1948, a doctor developed a cream that prevented bacteria from forming on the eye wounds of injured soldiers. After use, many of the soldiers reported a lengthening and thickening of their eyelashes. Talika harnessed the power found in that doctor's anti-bacterial cream to provide consumers with an easy-to-use eyelash treatment.

# How to Grow Thicker, Longer Lashes with Peptides

The secret ingredients in many of these eyelash products are peptides. Also used in anti-aging products, peptides have been found to reverse many of the aging processes that affect our appearance, including those that adversely impact the lash line.

**Jan Marini** — Jan Marini was one of the first companies to recognize the benefits of peptides in lash enhancement products. Jan Marini Lash uses a variety of ingredients, including peptides, to produce dense, gorgeous eyelashes. The Jan Marini product can also be used on the eyebrows with a similar effect. The product is applied with a mascara brush, and results are seen within a few weeks. Jan Marini Lash has been highly touted, and a multitude of customers are now enjoying positive results from the product.

**B. Kamins** — B. Kamins is another company that has produced an eyelash-enhancement product containing peptides, natural plant extracts, and a variety of vitamins. B. Kamins' conditioning agents keep existing lashes strong and healthy while peptides stimulate the growth of new lashes for a thicker appearance.

The B. Kamins product is promoted as a lash conditioner that generates stronger, more fortified lashes and provides the appearance of a fuller eye. According to B. Kamins, users can expect to see positive results within six to eight weeks.

**Neova** — Neova has jumped onto the lash enhancement bandwagon with stellar results. Neova Advanced Essential Lash is an eyelash conditioner with peptides, only this formula specifically uses copper peptides to achieve the desired results. Neova's copper peptides are relatively new to the skincare industry, but the results seen in anti-aging products have been impressive. This particular Neova product stimulates hair follicles directly to promote new eyelash growth for a fuller look.

If you want thicker, sexier eyelashes, you now have a number of options from which to choose. These new products provide the longer, thicker lashes you desire without surgery or prescription medication.

## ◈ LIP CONDITIONS AND LIP REPAIR

Full, pouty lips are the hallmark of some of the world's most beautiful celebrities. While some people are simply born with the kind of lips most women wish they had, many others need a little assistance in achieving that plump, sensual mouth. As the cosmetics industry has evolved, we have seen a plethora of lip products appear on the market that all claim to make lips fuller and plumper. There are also advanced lip products formulated to correct or repair damaged lips. Whether lips have been damaged by environmental factors or are the result of an inherent skin condition, lip repair products claim they can help.

When it comes to skincare, our lips are frequently the most neglected part of our face, even though they actually need the most care. Our lips contain just three to five cellular layers of skin, which makes them much thinner than facial skin. This means they are more sensitive to weather and other environmental conditions and to changes in our health. It's also why most experts recommend implementing a regular routine of lip treatment—one as simple as keeping your lips hydrated or as complex as major lip repair. It's easy to include lip enhancement in your skincare regimen given all the combination products on the market today.

Because they are sensitive, lips tend to dry out and chap more easily than the rest of your face. This is because the lips don't have sweat glands to create an extra layer of protection. This renders the lips vulnerable to damage from the environment, and more susceptible to the effects of aging, thus resulting in a variety of undesirable conditions. Lips tend to wrinkle faster, like the sensitive areas around the eyes. They also tend to lose their fullness, because the collagen that is imbedded deep in the layers tends to break down faster in the lips than in other areas of the face. Lip treatment, in most cases, involves stimulating collagen production to reverse the effects of time on collagen fibers underneath the skin.

One of the most common lip conditions, second only to the natural process of aging, is sun damage. People with lighter skin tones have significantly less melanin pigment in their lips than in their facial skin. This means that blood vessels appear closer to the surface, giving lips a pinkish or red color. Melanin is the pigment that helps screen out damaging UV rays. Without this protection, lips are at high risk for sunburn. UV rays can alter the appearance of lips as easily as they can cause premature aging on the face. The sun can also affect the levels of collagen within the lips, diminishing their natural resilience. The thin cellular layers may be eroded, damaged, or dried out due to UV rays, so wrinkles form more easily around the mouth and lip area, leading to premature aging.

Effective lip repair often includes lip treatments with sun protection, in addition to collagen restoration and hydration. With additional antioxidant support, good lip treatment products can provide a lip repair regimen that sets your lips on a path to a more youthful, healthier appearance. Most of these lip treatment products are as easy to use as lip gloss. The ones designed to be applied and worn throughout the day usually have a higher level of sunscreen protection—some are formulated to be worn under lipstick or gloss, and some for use alone. There are also many lip repair products designed to be worn overnight; they are specifically intended to increase hydration and restoration of lip cells.

## About Lip Plumpers and Enhancers

Lip plumpers or lip enhancers fall into a unique category of cosmetics. They're designed to make lips appear fuller and can be translucent, opaque, or tinted. While some lip enhancers are formulated primarily for the purpose of plumping, others are formulated to also repair damage, provide sunscreen benefits, and act as an anti-aging treatment to reduce fine lines and wrinkles on and around the lips.

Some lip plumpers can be worn alone as a lip gloss. From light shades to bright, colorful shades and glittery finishes, a wide range of looks can be achieved. The sheerer lip plumpers or lip enhancers are generally designed to be applied under lipstick.

Currently, the most popular lip plumper and lip enhancer brands on the market include LipFusion, ColoreScience, and Janson Beckett. However, almost every anti-aging skincare line on the market features lip plumpers or lip enhancer products. For instance, popular and trusted brands like BioElements, Borba, Decleor, and Dermalogica all have lip plumping and lip enhancing glosses, balms, and complexes. In fact, the majority of the products that fall into this latter group tend to be designed with more than just lip plumping in mind. Borba has a product called Cashmere Fiber Lip Kit that is formulated with cashmere fibers and shea butter to soften lips while providing protection. On the other hand, a brand like ColoreScience, which has a very wide range of lip plumpers and lip enhancers, has created kits to plump and enhance lips in more than one way. The ColoreScience Lip Restoration System includes a Crystalscience Lip Serum, a Lip Polish, and a Lip Exfoliator.

So how does a lip plumper make lips fuller and poutier? Lip plumpers contain ingredients like menthol or camphor that stimulate the delicate skin on the lips and make them swell slightly. This is often enough of a plumping effect to reduce fine lines and wrinkles as well. Blends of antioxidants like vitamin C help hydrate the lips while increasing plumpness. Additional specially formulated blends help stimulate new cell growth and enhance lip color, while others repair and restore skin. Dermalogica's AGE Smart Renewal Lip Complex uses a patented polypeptide technology to repair and restore skin.

# ❧ 3 ❧

# SCIENCE, TECHNOLOGY AND ANTI-AGING SKINCARE

There are many skincare techniques that individuals can use to manage wrinkles, lines, sagging skin, and other imperfections and signs of aging. These may include laser techniques, dermabrasion, chemical peels, and creams containing retinol, peptides, stem cells, and other ingredients discovered within the past twenty years. Recently, however, science and research have played an even more important role in the development of anti-aging skincare products. As new technologies become available, skincare researchers explore how to take advantage of those innovations in the dermatological sector. With new gene expression discoveries and other innovations, the field of anti-aging techniques has made huge leaps in giving people the ability to enhance their appearances, enabling them to look and feel years younger, and teaching them how to prevent and successfully treat skin disorders or imperfections.

Without these scientific advances and the research performed to prove the effectiveness and safety of these new methods, important anti-aging skincare products and procedures may never have come to light. Skincare research is constantly evolving, and results are shared with other professionals through scientific publications like the Journal of Dermatology. These scientists also present their experimental findings at conferences organized by prestigious institutions like The American Academy of Dermatology.

The science involved in developing anti-aging skincare products and techniques, particularly those related to DNA, stem cells, liposomes, and nanotechnology, is fascinating and a sign of how far we have advanced in the field of skincare. In the past, only laser treatments, retinol creams, or other, more aggressive treatments were effective for skin disorders such as severe sun damage. Now, new advances in stem cell research have produced a number of skincare and anti-aging products in the forms of lotions, creams, serums, and sunscreens that contain stem cell repair ingredients.

Anti-oxidants can help with the loss of collagen and are quicker and longer lasting when combined with increasingly new and effective technology, such as liposomes and nanotechnology. Peptides can also boost collagen production. When used in conjunction with new ingredient delivery systems, these substances work much more effectively since they can now penetrate the skin's outer dermal layer, affect the skin's cells, and produce new collagen.

Consumers are more educated today than ever before, and they know if they are being scammed. This new breed of consumer looks to companies that perform diligent research and conduct safe, clinical trials for information. Consumers don't want products that might cause harm to people, animals, or the environment during the course of research, development, or production.

Fortunately, the new science of skincare is making the grade. Consumer satisfaction is sure to grow when people explore what is available from a scientific point of view. These products deliver on their promises to restore damaged skin and to minimize or eliminate the signs of aging.

The public's continued interest in and commitment to health and wellness education and concern for beauty will be instrumental in generating more research, more innovative development, and newer products for skin protection.

## ❖ THE DNA IN YOUR SKIN

Research and testing have allowed scientists to discover single nucleotide polymorphisms in our skin that helps us to evaluate overall skin health. Working with this technology, companies now have a host of DNA skincare products that specifically address aging, wrinkling, and damage caused by the sun and environmental hazards.

DNA skincare products are constantly being researched, and new developments are continuously implemented. These products are tested for UV protection capabilities, and for their ability to protect skin under all kinds of environmental assaults. They are tested for quality, purity, effectiveness, and performance. These products are formulated based on leading research from around the globe, and using information about mitochondria DNA and molecular skin structure.

DNA products can be created for individual clients in special spa-type salons or clinics after a skin test is performed. The skin test involves taking a cell sample from inside the mouth and sending it away for analysis. A highly trained technician or physician will then make recommendations for skincare products based on the individual's DNA results.

Other DNA-based skincare products can be purchased with just a general assessment of your skin's state of health (e.g., anti-wrinkling for women over 40). DNA specific skincare products can be generically made for wrinkles, anti-aging, rejuvenation of dull skin, and to address specific areas.

Wilma Schumann's DNA Plus is an excellent example of a product for consumers looking for the best skincare available. Products like this use science and technology to create skincare lines for cleansing, moisturizing, acne care, anti-aging, anti-wrinkling, toning, and fine tuning the pigment of the skin, face, lips, and eyes.

## ◈ STEM CELLS

Stem cells are found in all multi-celled organisms. Through mitosis, they divide and transform into specialized cell types and repair systems in the body. During the early stages of life, a stem cell has the potential to form itself into different cell types inside the body. In certain organs, such as the intestines and bone marrow, stem cells can divide over and over again to repair and/or replace damaged tissue. Research scientists now use stem cells to test new drugs or medicines and to develop models that are used to study normal development in the body.

Stem cells can also be directed to develop into new and specific cell types. This gives scientists the ability to replace cells and tissues. Besides allowing scientists to treat conditions such as spinal cord injury, stroke, or Alzheimer's, stem cells can also treat skin disorders, such as burns, using stem cells from plants like roses. These stem cell-stimulating technologies can also be very effective for anti-aging skincare.

## PhytoCellTec™ Malus Domestica

PhytoCellTec™ uses stem cells from a rare Swiss apple famed for its longevity to improve the longevity of human skin cells, protect the skin from UV damage, and support genes that repair DNA. This anti-wrinkle treatment was evaluated in a study of 20 volunteers between the ages of 37 and 64. The cream was applied twice daily to the crows feet around the volunteers' eyes. 100% of the participants saw a significant and visible decrease in wrinkle depth by the conclusion of the study.

Ageless Derma used this technology to formulate Ageless Derma Stem Cell and Peptide Anti wrinkle Cream

Lysolecithin stimulates keratinocyte stem cells found in the outer layer of the skin. This helps them to produce energy and enhances enzyme production, which leads to the production of new skin. Ingredients such as retinyl ester lipopeptides regenerate epidermal (outer skin) stem cells, helping to repair DNA damage by metabolizing positive genes. Flaxeedoyl can augment the antioxidant response, which stimulates the renewal of cells.

Stem cell technologies focus on polypeptides and enzymes to regenerate the body's own epidermal stem cells. Actual stem cells are not rubbed onto the skin with these products; the body's own skin stem cells are activated and renewed. The enzymes and polypeptides used in the product renew the skin and make the user look younger.

Stem cell-stimulating products and techniques aid the skin in absorbing appropriate ingredients and help diminish facial lines and wrinkles.

Stem cells taken from fat tissue, developed into a cosmetic serum and smoothed on the skin stimulate collagen production. This helps lift and support sagging skin. They also help the skin to retain its natural moisture, making the user look brighter and younger. Wrinkle filler can be added to the mix to erase crow's-feet, laugh lines and frown lines.

Stem cell techniques offer a natural way to look younger without the need for dangerous chemicals, needles, or surgery. If the skin is inflamed, stem cell products combat the inflammation and protect the skin from ultraviolet radiation. Because they also fight against damaging free radicals, stem cell regeneration products can help prevent skin pigment discoloration and collagen loss.

## ❖ FETAL CELLS IN SKINCARE

Scientific research conducted by physicians and scientists in various laboratories around the world has proved that there are healing properties in fetal cells for restoring and slowing the aging process of the skin. Cell banks have been established to provide fetal cells from scrapings, so there is a nearly endless supply available for research and the development of skincare products.

Through years of research, physicians have discovered that fetal skin cells have the unique ability to heal wounds without scarring. Switzerland created a biotechnology process to extract the rich proteins responsible for scar-less wound healing from cultured fetal skin cells. The products developed by Neocutis, including PSP, are the newest, most cutting-edge cosmaceuticals in the marketplace.

**Note:** The technology using fetal skin cells is still very controversial in the skincare industry.

## ❖ NANOTECHNOLOGY

The term *nanotechnology* refers to the ability to handle matter that is very small in scale—about the size of molecules or atoms. The new and innovative materials being developed with nanotechnology have a wide spectrum of applications; for instance, nanotechnology is utilized in medicine to produce energy, electronics, and biomaterials. In essence, any technique or tool that is small enough can be referred to as nanotechnology. Scientists can build working systems that are remarkably light, strong, intelligent, and durable if they have the control and the ability to change matter on the scale of nanometers.

Speaking at the 68th annual meeting of the American Academy of Dermatology, Adnan Nasir (MD, PhD, and FAAD), the clinical assistant professor in the Department of Dermatology at the University of North Carolina, presented an overview of nanotechnology and how nanoparticles may eventually be used in cosmetic products.

According to Dr. Nasir, "Research in the area of nanotechnology has increased significantly over the years, and I think there will be considerable growth in this area in the near future. The challenge is that there is no standard at this time to evaluate the safety and efficacy of topical products that contain nanosized particles."

With the aid of nanotechnology, skincare products can better penetrate beneath the skin's surface, allowing them to target specific areas. Skincare products that use nanotechnology to convert ingredients into nanosized elements improve the blood's circulation and in the process reduce dark circles under the eyes by eliminating the waste products and oxidized particles that cause the dark circles in the first place.

Nanotechnology can also be used for other pigmentation issues. Combining vitamin K with nanotechnology alleviates the appearance of unsightly spider veins. While vitamin K has been used to treat spider veins in the past, it can only sufficiently penetrate the skin for a good effect through the use of nanotechnology.

People that want the wrinkles and lines removed from their lips no longer have to undergo lip augmentation. Through nanotechnology, the fullness of the lips can be increased with lipstick containing plumper ingredients. Stretch marks, scars, and sagging skin can also be helped with nanotechnology.

The microscopic particles used in nanotechnological skincare treatments can penetrate the skin—absorption is quick. Skincare products, such as anti-aging creams and sunscreen, can now be manufactured as nano skincare products to increase their effectiveness. The primary benefit of using nanoparticles in sunscreens is that the particles can enter all the tiny pits and cracks of the skin, giving protection that is more evenly distributed on the skin's surface. Sunscreen products that use nanoparticles are more cosmetically appealing because they seem to vanish into the skin when applied. This leads people to use them more frequently and consistently, contributing to the positive anti-aging effects attributed to the product. Sunscreens using *macro-sized* particles actually absorb ultraviolet light and can be toxic to human, whereas sunscreens containing nanoparticles prevent ultraviolet absorption. Products that use nanotechnology are considered natural products. The products do not simply coat the skin's surface; they penetrate—an advancement that has been a long time coming.

## ◆ LIPOSOMES

Liposomes are structures composed of phospholipids, the same materials found in cell membranes. Phospholipids' heads are attracted to water while their tails are repelled by water, creating a bilayer which can be used to artificially build liposomes. The word liposome literally derives from the Greek words *fat* and *body*. Liposomes were developed by Dr. Bangham in 1965, to transport drugs, vaccines, and other materials directly to the body site where they were needed. Liposomes can be used in the same way to carry cosmetics to the skin. The first cosmetics containing liposomes were developed in 1986; now they are commonplace in hundreds of gels, creams, and moisturizers.

Using liposomes to deliver cosmetic ingredients increases the penetration and diffusion of the active ingredients and allows the substances to be more selectively transported to the target areas. Release time is also spread out, making the cosmetics last longer. These substances have greater stability and there are few, if any, negative side effects.

When a gel or cream containing liposomes is smoothed on the skin's surface, the liposomes merge with cell membranes and release active substances into the target cells. The effectiveness of the liposomes depends on the size used. Generally, the smaller the liposomes, the more deeply they penetrate and the longer the active ingredients last.

Liposomes can be added to moisturizers to ensure good hydration. The phospholipids used in the construction of liposomes contain moisture and encourage the ingredients to better adhere to the skin, hydrating it. Liposomes also create a barrier on the skin's surface, trapping moisture underneath the lipid's membrane. This hydrates the skin's layers and repels other substances such as sunlight or sweat.

Some anti-wrinkle creams utilize liposomes in combination with vitamins A and E, avocado, shea butter, or soya. The gels are usually light and soft on the skin and help diminish crow's-feet and fine lines. Gels using the liposome delivery system are soothing as they bind in moisture and lubricate skin tissues.

## ◈ GENOMA

By working with modern genetic information, skincare research has made great strides in the past few decades. A genoma is the ordered set of genetic material that makes up a living organism. Scientists completed the ordering of the human genome in 2003, ushering in the post-genoma era and bringing even more exciting innovations to the skincare industry.

When the genoma sequence for Malassezia globosa (M. globosa) was completed, innovations in dandruff and dry skin conditions began to evolve. M. globosa is a yeast fungus found naturally in living cells that can cause dandruff and other severe dry skin conditions. DNA sequencing technologies have helped scientists learn much more about these conditions than ever before.

Now, with DNA microarrays, researchers working on the production of new skincare products can determine the gene expression of an entire human genome, all at once. Different skincare products can be more accurately compared and assessed by using DNA microarrays. The variations of gene expression produced by a peptide, or any biologically active substance, provide us with new and significant information on the effect a given substance has on skin tissue.

DNA microarray techniques have spurred the invention and production of new products and therapies that can reduce the appearance of fine lines and wrinkles while also improving the tone and clarity of the skin. DNA microarrays are also useful in understanding abnormal scarring. In the future this could help in the repair processes of both normal and abnormal wounds.

## ❖ NEW AND INNOVATIVE PRODUCTS AND INGREDIENTS

### Vialox

Vialox is an anti-wrinkle ingredient that is very potent. It comes in powder form and has been proven to reduce wrinkling—through the contraction of muscle cells—by 49%. It is similar to Botox, but it is a topical cream rather than an injection, making it attractive to people reluctant to try facial injections.

Vialox produces a Botox-like reduction in wrinkles. In clinical studies, volunteers applied Vialox to one half of their faces twice a day for 28 days. The subjects were women between the ages of thirty and sixty. The primary purpose of the study was to determine the effectiveness of Vialox on crow's-feet— but it was discovered to be equally effective on other facial wrinkles as well.

Vialox is composed of a pentapeptide (pentapeptide-3) that relaxes muscles in the skin. Pentapeptide-3 is manufactured by a Swiss pharmaceutical company. It works by blocking nerves in the postsynaptic membrane and then binds to specific receptors in the nerve, preventing sodium ions from being released. This stops the electric charge in the nerve (known as depolarization) which would otherwise cause wrinkles. Vialox is very similar to curare, the poison used by some South American tribes for blow darts.

The Vialox powder kit is sold in two vials—one contains penpeptide-3 in powder form, while the second contains a solvent that dissolves the powder. The purpose of the two-vial packaging is to keep the active ingredient fresh for as long as possible.

Only one or two drops of Vialox, smoothed into the face, are needed to address crow's-feet, wrinkles on the forehead, frown lines, and nasolabial folds. Results can be seen within a month. The product lasts up to two weeks after mixing. Apply Vialox twice daily for the first month, and then maintain the positive effects with a daily application thereafter. A 14-day supply of Relax Plus Vialox sells for about forty-two dollars.

## Revinage

Revinage is made from a retinoid-like vegetable source that offers extra benefits for the skin. Retinoids are used as skin plumpers as they smooth and reduce wrinkles from inside the skin. They help stimulate collagen production and rejuvenate the skin, adding renewed elasticity.

Natural retinoids are derived from vitamin A, a substance contained in plant materials. They work to unclog pores, increase collagen production, and erase fine lines within just a few weeks' time. Synthetic retinoids are very similar to natural retinoids. They activate retinoic acid receptors (RARs) in the skin. This helps trigger plumping, wrinkle smoothing, and lightening of the skin.

However, retinoids can sometimes be irritating to the skin. Revinage is formulated to eliminate this type of reaction by targeting only the RARs that are necessary to produce the desired effect. Most synthetic retinoids can be used in direct sunlight, while true retinoids cannot. While using a retinoid, such as Retin-A, you must apply a sunscreen to avoid sunburn or skin damage. (You may want to wear sunscreen even with synthetic retinoids just to ensure that there is no toxicity and that the retinoids remain stable in the sunlight.)

Revinage decreases wrinkles and lightens the skin by reducing melanin production. It can also control oil production, resulting in fewer acne breakouts. Revinage also acts as an anti-inflammatory agent with anti-oxidant effects.

## PhytoCellTec

PhytoCellTec is a technology developed by Mibelle Biochemistry that protects skin stem cells. It is derived from the stem cells of a Swiss apple tree, which produces apples famous for their longevity which are rich in phytonutrients and suffer little shriveling over time. The plant's stem cells are obtained using PhytoCellTec's technology and placed into cosmetic skincare products to guarantee that skin cells live longer with less wrinkling. This technology helps protect human skin cells, slowing the aging process and minimizing wrinkling of the skin.

The skin creams made with PhytoCellTec are enhanced through the addition of vitamins C and E.

The actual PhytoCellTec process intentionally damages a tiny piece of the plant material in order to induce calluses. These calluses are incubated on slide plates and, when developed, are harvested in order to obtain stem cells. These stem cells are then processed, captured, and placed into liposomes.

## Melanostatin 5

Melanostatin 5 (or nonoapeptide-1) is a synthesized peptide used in cosmetic products to rid the skin of abnormal pigmentation, reduce wrinkles, and smooth the skin's surface.

Peptides are strings of amino acids, the building blocks of life. When applied to the skin in the form of creams or lotions, synthesized peptides act as messengers to skin cell receptors, telling them how to react.

Melanostatin 5 is a synthesized peptide that works by stopping the melanocyte hormone that is stimulated by UV light. Melanostatin 5 instructs the melanocytes to stop producing melanin. This can lighten the skin's pigmentation or prevent hyper-pigmentation. When included in anti-aging products, Melanostatin 5 can also help lighten dark circles under the eyes. The ingredient delivers very positive effects within four to twelve weeks when used in cosmetic creams and lotions. It lightens the skin by at least 33% with the initial application. Over time, and with continued use, that percentage increases.

This is a safe lightening ingredient that is quite effective and reliable. Products containing Melanostatin 5 do take time to work, but once they have taken effect, the results are usually very good. However, it is not a permanent solution to hyper-pigmentation. If a client stops using the cream or lotion, the product ceases to work and results fade.

Products should contain a high percentage of Melanostatin 5 in order to guarantee positive results. A minimum of 2–4% of the cream is the norm. Complimentary ingredients should also be present for the best outcomes. Ingredients such as (5%) Matrixl, (10%) Argireline, (3%) Rigin, (3%) Eyeliss and (5%) Regu-age are excellent additions. When you read the product label, look for higher percentages of each substance to achieve the best results.

With the addition of Melanostatin 5, skincare products lighten age spots, freckles, and melasma. They work in anti-aging creams to help brighten skin damaged by the sun, even out blotchiness, and firm the skin at the cellular level.

## Matrixyl 3000

Matrixyl 3000, developed by the Sederma Corporation, is made up of two matrikines peptides, Pal-GHK (palmitoyl oligopeptide) and Pal-GQPR (palmitoyl tetrapeptide-7). These work together as antioxidants to fight the damaging effects of aging on the skin. Together they stimulate the matrix molecules (collagens and fibronectin) and enable Matrixyl 3000 to reduce wrinkles. Matrixyl 3000 is a white gel with a pH between 4.0 and 6.0, and a water content of 30%.

Pal-GHK is a short chain of three amino acids that are connected to palmitic acid, a fatty acid that improves the chain's oil solubility and skin penetration. It is a collagen molecule that detects any decline in the skin matrix. GHK stimulates new collagen synthesis.

The other component of Matrixyl 3000, Pal-GQPR, is a short chain of four amino acids that is also connected to palmitic acid and works similarly to the Pal-GHK above. It also reduces interleukin-6 production, keratinocytes, and fibroblasts. This substance won't promote inflammation or degrading of the skin matrix, either of which can lead to wrinkles and sagging. Pal-GQPR may help slow the decline of the skin matrix and stimulate the growth of new cells.

The addition of Matrixyl 3000 to cosmetic skincare products reduces wrinkles and improves the skin's elasticity and tone. As an anti-wrinkle ingredient, Matrixyl reduces the density and volume of wrinkles and minimizes sagging of the neck and facial skin. Studies have shown that Matrixyl 3000 reduces wrinkle density by 33%, lessens wrinkle volume by 23%, and decreases wrinkle depth by 20%.

Matrixyl 3000 helps rejuvenate the skin's dermal area, thereby fighting wrinkles. This ingredient helps stimulate collagen production, which in turn helps to produce a more even and luminous skin tone while increasing the thickness of the skin's outer layer. The creams formulated with Matrixyl 3000 penetrate deeply into the skin where they can retain the moisture the skin needs.

This ingredient also aids in fighting free radicals, in evening skin tones, increasing skin's thickness, keeping moisture in and making the skin feel firmer and healthier. In addition to Matrixyl 3000, some cosmetic skin products include other antioxidants such as copper peptides, marine collagen, grape, tea, and/or algae.

## Darkout

Darkout is useful for people with uneven skin tones, no matter what their ethnicity. When added to face creams, body lotions, hand creams, and anti-aging creams, it cures blotchiness, sun damage, hormonal damage, scarring, and the effects of aging. Skin color changes may be the result of anything from smoking, to genetics, to emotional stress, in addition to the causes mentioned above.

Skin cosmetics containing the ingredient Darkout give the skin a radiant, luminous appearance. It evens skin pigmentation, helps to fade age spots and wrinkles, and helps with hyper-pigmentation (when an area of the skin darkens due to an increase in melanin production). Hyper-pigmentation can occur in the epidermis, the dermis, or occasionally in both areas. An increase in melanin production can be caused by overexposure to the sun, inflammation of the skin tissue, or any other skin damage such as acne scarring. People with darker skin colors are more likely to have hyper-pigmentation issues, particularly if they spend a lot of time in the sun.

There are various types of hyper-pigmentation. Melasma presents as dark brown patches on the face — particularly the forehead, temples and cheeks. It is usually found in pregnant women or women taking birth control pills. About ten percent of the time, it may also be seen in women who are not pregnant or in men. All of these patients, however, have melasma due to sun exposure. Melasma does fade in women, but rarely fades in men.

Lentigines are brown, oval-shaped spots caused by repeated sun exposure. They are also known as liver spots (solar lentigines). Usually found on the face and hands, they begin to appear around middle-age and increase as people get older. Age spots may be associated with melanoma or skin cancer. Some hyper-pigmentations may be due to drug use or disease.

Darkout is a naturally-derived product, made up of African star grass roots called *corms*. It works by inhibiting tyrosinase, reducing the synthesis of melanin.

# Argireline

Argireline is an ingredient used in some anti-wrinkle cosmetic products. These products are applied directly to the skin. Argireline is actually the trademark name for acetyl hexapeptide-3, a molecule that is part of a peptide chain. Argireline is made up of a chain of six amino acids or proteins and so is shorter than a Botox string.

Argireline helps erase deep creases, wrinkles, and lines around the forehead and the eyes, like those found in crow's-feet. When Argireline is added to a chemically-made cosmetic compound, it relaxes the muscles that cause the face to smile, frown, or make other expressions. Its function is very similar to that of Botox. By relaxing tension on the face, lines and wrinkles are much less likely to form in the first place. Neurotransmitters in the brain tell our facial muscles to tense in certain situations; Argireline inhibits these neurotransmitters, allowing the muscles to relax. When this ingredient is combined with other cosmetic components, it makes a wonderful, moisturizing, anti-aging, skin-resurfacing product.

Clinical experiments have shown that creams containing 10% Argireline reduced the depth of wrinkles in 27% of the women tested. Even with lower concentrations of the ingredient (5%), women still saw a 17% reduction in lines and creases.

# Axolight

Axolight is an active ingredient contained in products that lighten the skin. It is a chemical structure composed of ArabinoXylo-Oligosaccharides. It works by inhibiting melanogenesis (a process that causes the cells to produce melanin—the pigment that gives our skin, eyes, and hair their unique colors).

Melanogenesis also causes us to tan when we are out in the sunlight, especially those of us with lighter skin. People with very fair skin may burn when exposed to the sun due to melanogenesis. By including Axolight as an active ingredient in skincare products, melanogenesis is inhibited and causes less damage to the skin. Axolight can specifically inhibit the tyrosinase-related protein enzyme needed to activate tyrosinase—this limits melanogenesis at different levels and reduces skin pigmentation.

Aging, the sun's rays, and stress all have negative effects on our skin. Axolight can reduce these effects by preventing age spots and other types of damage. It can lighten skin, and allow the cream you've applied to work longer after sun exposure. It has proven very successful for all-over sun care, including the hands and the face, prior to, during, and after exposure.

In one clinical test, a cream containing 3% Axolight was smoothed on a woman's skin every other day. She was then exposed to the sun's UV rays daily for ten days. Her results showed that melanogenesis was reduced by 88%.

In other experiments, Axolight was compared with creams containing Arbutin, a skin lightening cream. Of the control group using Axolight cream, 91% of the people showed a lightened effect on their skin, while only 82% of those using Arbutin exhibited a similar lightening effect. Axolight cream worked more quickly than the Arbutin cream.

Cosmetically, Axolight is useful for lightening the skin; when included in anti-aging creams, it addresses age spots.

## ℬ 4 ℭ

# KNOW THE SKIN YOU ARE IN

B elieve it or not, most people have no idea what their skin type is. Some may be able to guess, but few will be able to tell you with certainty.

We all fall into four categories when it comes to skin type: oily, dry, a combination of oily and dry, or normal. Knowing your skin type is very important. This is how you're able to purchase the correct makeup and skincare products. The last thing you want is to put the wrong products on your face. In order to avoid mistakes, here a few things you should look for when determining your skin type and how it is best treated.

## Oily Skin

Your skin falls in the category of oily if you find that it always looks shiny. The area that seems to be most affected is called the T-zone. This area is formed by the width of your forehead and then from the center of your forehead straight down to the tip of your nose. If this area is always shiny, chances are you have oily skin. Another way to determine if you have oily skin is to spend some time simply examining your pores. Large pores are an indication that you have oily skin. Your makeup offers another clue to your skin type. If you have oily skin, foundation tends to migrate; it may gather in wrinkles on the forehead or in the creases around the mouth.

People with oily skin should look for cleansing products that are oil-free. The last thing your skin needs is more oil. A very important step in cleaning an oily face is the application of toner. Toners help clear away makeup and dirt that may have been left behind by the cleanser. After cleansing and toning, you need to moisturize. Water-based moisturizers are the best choice for oily skin.

## Dry / Sensitive Skin

When identifying dry skin, look for flakes. Dry skin tends to be flaky, especially around the eyebrows and nose. Unlike oily skin, dry skin is associated with very small pores, which is why moisturizing is very important. The texture is another way to detect dry skin. If the surface of the skin has a rough feel, or it is tight and itchy, your skin is probably dry. The itching and tightness may be more noticeable after you've cleaned your face. Dry skin tends to be more sensitive than oily and combination skin. If you have skin that's very sensitive to the sun, wind, or cold, it is probably in the dry category.

Contrary to popular belief, dry skin is not caused by a lack of oil; it's actually caused by lack of water, so the key is to look for ways to add more water to the skin. Look for cleansing products that are specifically made for dry skin. You'll find that many of these products are water-based. Dry skin needs to be kept moisturized at all times.

Sensitive skin requires special care. There are many ingredients in products that produce dryness, itchiness, and sometimes even a rash or other types of visible irritation. Most people with sensitive skin feel that their cosmetics and skincare product choices are limited. However, there are several cosmetic companies that specialize in products designed specifically for people with sensitive skin or allergies. Consumers with sensitive skin should be sure to investigate the specific ingredients in products before purchasing, as even some of those that claim to be safe for sensitive skin can cause irritation.

## Combination Skin

This is actually the most common skin type. Combination skin has characteristics of both oily and dry skin. You'll find that your face is oily in some places, usually around the T-zone, and dry around the cheeks. If you've found that skin products work well on part of your skin but irritate other parts, that's usually a good indication that you have combination skin.

Caring for combination skin is difficult because your skin is both dry and oily. The good news is that there is help for combination skin. The key is to choose a mild cleanser. Use the cleanser on the entire face at least twice a day. After cleansing, choose a good moisturizer and use it on the dry areas of your face.

## Normal Skin

Normal skin is just what its name suggests—normal. There is no flaking or excessive oil present on the skin. Instead, the skin has a very smooth texture. Not many people are fortunate enough to have normal skin, but if you're one of the few, consider yourself very lucky.

Even if your skin type is normal, it's still important to keep it well-cleansed. Choose a cleanser specifically for normal skin, and use it twice a day, in the morning and again at night. Use a light moisturizer after cleaning. To keep your skin looking great, protect it from the sun with sunscreen. Monitor what you eat and drink. If you're fortunate enough to have normal skin, you want to do everything in your power to keep it that way.

### ◈ Managing Your Dry Skin

Dry skin is problematic, physically and socially. Dry skin can be irritable, uncomfortable, and have long-term detrimental effects on the condition and appearance of your face. Dry and flaking skin can also lead to a lack of confidence in social situations.

Dry skin can take many forms. Most people experience slightly dry skin at some time, whether through sunburn or contact with harsh chemicals. A hormone imbalance can lead to dry skin, and allergic reactions may cause the skin to shed or suffer cellular damage. Other medical conditions, like dermatitis and eczema, also cause the skin to itch, flake, and become sore.

Sun-damaged skin may become dry and loose due to a lack of hydration and the loss of elasticity. When this happens, cellular turnover slows down, and cells become damaged and begin to flake. The epidermis is fragile and needs to be protected. Thankfully, there have been a number of advances in skincare incorporating ingredients that aid dry skin.

## How to Hydrate Dry Skin

Skin hydration is essential to prevent dry skin. There are many ways to help hydrate your skin. For example, drinking eight glasses of water a day keeps the dermis and epidermis hydrated and energized.

Moisturizing daily with an effective skincare product also helps prevent dry skin. Applying medicated moisturizers to eczema-affected skin can help prevent stress-induced irritation and soreness. Becoming educated about dry skin is the first step toward prevention.

**B. Kemis Antipruritic Cream** helps aid many different dry skin related problems, including eczema, allergic reactions, and dermatitis. This is not a prescription cream, nor does it highly medicate the skin. It will, however, effectively sooth dry skin.

**Bioelements Absolute Moisture** is a non-comedogenic moisturizer that permits self-adjusting hydration for dry and combination skin. It contains Sodium PCA, which is an effective skin softener, as well as other moisture-bonding ingredients to hold moisture in and keep skin-drying elements out.

If moisturizing is already part of your daily routine, and if you suffer from dry skin, why not invest in a facial moisturizer or cream that replenishes dehydrated skin cells? Preventing and healing dry skin has been made simple. Using effective, scientifically-formulated skincare products will protect your face and keep it youthful.

## Check the Products You Are Using

Very often soaps or other cleansers contribute to dry skin. These products contain ingredients that are too harsh; you need something milder that cleanses the skin without robbing it of essential oils. The best product to use on dry skin is a mild cleanser, because, even when unscented, soaps often have perfumes in them. Check product labels very carefully and ask your skincare professional for advice in finding the right products for you.

Do not use abrasive brushes or sponges to cleanse the skin. Most people's skin cannot tolerate these implements as they strip away important natural oils. Try to avoid rough, itchy clothing (e.g. unlined wool) that can irritate the skin.

Medications like diuretics or acne treatments can have a dehydrating effect on the skin. When your doctor prescribes a medication, be sure to ask if it will lead to dry skin. Always ask for medications or products made specifically for people with dry or sensitive skin. There are many products available on the market today; finding alternatives for those that are too harsh should be a simple matter.

## ◈ Managing Your Oily Skin

There are a number of ways that cosmetic companies try to gain a competitive edge for oily skincare treatment. One of the most common strategies is for companies to compete against each other to provide you with the absolute best products available on the market. Amazingly enough, this global company vs. company competition has been the catalyst for the creation of several fabulous oily skincare products. However, although there are thousands of products that promise to eliminate oily skin, very few actually live up to their promises to provide long-term results. Here are a few suggestions for products that have proven successful for oily skin treatment.

**Astara Blue Flame Oil-Free Moisturizer** provides oily skin with the proper moisture balance while controlling excess oil and preventing clogged pores.

**B. Kamins Oily to Normal Starter Kit** offers a complete line of products that work to balance the skin, leaving it fresh and oil-free.

**DermaNew Microdermabrasion Acne & Oily Clarifying System** is designed to provide your skin with a gentle, yet thorough, resurfacing. Able to polish and refine as it treats, this product has the power to decongest the surface of the skin as it diminishes the appearance of post-breakout discoloration. When used regularly, this powerful product has the capacity to prevent future breakouts.

**Glytone Normal to Oily Skin System Kit Step 1 with Mini Peel** is specially formulated for use on normal to oily skin types. This kit is ideal for gifting, traveling, or just stocking up on your favorite products. These products are enriched with small amounts of glycolic acid, an ingredient that works to smooth slight imperfections of the skin.

**Cellex-C Sea Silk Oil-Free Moisturizer 60mlC** — The primary benefit of this product is fresh, vibrant-looking skin that is soft to the touch. An excellent moisturizer for normal, combination, or oily skin, Cellex-C is potent enough to yield immediate results, yet is gentle enough for use on even the most sensitive skin. Effects are instantaneous, and they become even more apparent at the four to six-week mark. Cellex-C Sea Silk Oil-Free Moisturizer is appropriate for both men and women.

## ◈ Managing Your Sensitive Skin

People with sensitive skin (typically a genetic condition) have a very limited number of appropriate skincare products available to them. Sensitive skin frequently reacts adversely to makeup and other skincare products. Dryness, redness, blotchiness, burning sensations, and even the onset of adult acne may be caused by contact with products inappropriate for sensitive skin. Because of the high risk for rashes and other skin conditions common to people with sensitive skin, effective skincare products are often difficult to find.

**AminoGenesis Cocoon** is a hydrating moisturizer that provides a protective, preventative barrier against environmental assaults on the skin. This unique formula smoothes the skin, eliminates flakiness, and supplies a soft base for makeup. AminoGenesis moisturizer won't leave behind a greasy finish, and when blended with amino acids, it can actually heal the skin.

**BioElements Recovery Serum** is an excellent choice for sensitive skin that tends to be dry and itchy. This product restores the skin's natural moisture balance and soothes irritated skin. Because sensitive skin commonly has an adverse reaction to cosmetics, a mineral makeup is the perfect solution. Combining natural minerals and vitamins, these products, like those in the Ageless Derma

Mineral Makeup line, provide the skin with nutrients, without causing irritation.

# ɞ 5 ଔ

# ACNE

## ◈ ACNE FACTS: MORE THAN SKIN DEEP

A cne is one of the most common skin conditions, affecting up to 80% of the population in their teens, adults into their 40s, and pregnant women. It is generally exacerbated by oily skin, but no skin type is immune. Excess oil or debris clogs pores and generates blackheads and whiteheads or develops into cystic acne that becomes inflamed or infected. These cysts can rupture and cause scars.

The effects of blemishes—mild or extreme—can be more far-reaching than many people realize. From first impressions, to personal psychological issues, to your skin's health, acne is a significant challenge for many. Luckily, there's a wealth of information available about the subject and many options for treatments. When you understand what causes acne, and how your skin renews, you're on your way to addressing your specific skin problems.

Many things can cause acne. Some of the most common causes include genetics, your body's hormonal balance, changes in hormone levels, skin irritation, stress, hyperactive sebaceous glands, the accumulation of dead cells on the surface of the skin, bacteria in pores, use of certain medications, and even exposure to chemicals. Most types of acne are treatable.

## ◆ Acne Treatments: Ingredients in Popular Acne Treatments

There are many over-the-counter (OTC) acne cleansers, creams, lotions, gels, and solutions available. Some are designed to address existing skin blemishes, some to prevent them, and others to do both. There are *systems* which combine several products that work together as part of a regimen, and there are *acne zappers* or single purpose products designed to target specific blemishes.

The most popular acne treatments are designed to reduce the abnormal clumping of cells in follicles, help control increased oil production, manage and fight bacteria, and help reduce and mitigate inflammation. Not all treatments are effective, however. The ingredients they contain and the concentrations in which they're formulated are critical to the effectiveness of any given product. Some of the key ingredients effective in acne treatments include:

**Benzoyl peroxide**—This product destroys P. acnes bacteria while reducing oil production. It is a strong oxidizer and works well fighting bacteria. However, even as it helps your skin control oil production, it can lead to dryness, so when opting for acne treatments that contain this ingredient, make sure they also contain non-comedogenic moisturizers to counter the dryness.

**Resorcinol**—Unclogs pores to break down blackheads and whiteheads.

**Salicylic acid**—Works like resorcinol, but also helps keep the cells that line the hair follicles from shedding.

**Triclosan**—Its antibacterial properties control P. acnes levels.

**Sulfur**—Exfoliates to promote normal skin cell turnover while preventing clumping.

## ◈ Treating Acne at Home

If you struggle with acne, you are probably constantly trying to find a cure. You try product after product, but none of them seem to make a difference. You wash your face morning, noon, and night, and never fail to exfoliate or apply a deep-pore cleansing mask. You follow every acne-reducing tip you can find, which means that you have completely eliminated things like French fries and chocolate from your diet—yet, your acne remains. In fact, it may even appear to get worse.

Your frustration is easy to understand. Acne sufferers often perpetuate their problem without realizing it. Myths about the true causes of acne have resulted in a long list of *treatments* that serve no purpose, and may even cause harm.

Many people believe that acne is the result of dirty skin or poor hygiene. Not true. In fact, scrubbing and over cleansing the skin can actually cause acne to worsen because it irritates and dries the skin. If you are currently trying to scrub your acne away, stop it! There are multiple things that cause acne, but acne caused by bacteria and hormones is the most common form. Acne-causing bacteria live naturally on the skin's surface. The presence of bacteria is not a result of dirty skin. This bacterium is an irritant and converts the oil produced by your skin into substances that irritate the skin even further. Hormones that cause acne trigger oil glands to overproduce. The excess oil plugs the pores, resulting in acne.

The best way to treat acne at home may not be what you expect. The number one rule to observe when treating acne at home is to minimize irritation. Wash your face in the morning and in the evening with a mild cleanser and warm water. Find a cleanser that is specifically designed for acne, like B. Kamin's Hydrating Acne Wash. Next, apply a topical acne lotion. There are thousands of products on the market that claim to produce clear skin; however, the most effective acne lotions, like B. Kamin's Medicated Acne Gel, contain one of two key ingredients, **benzoyl peroxide** and/or **salicylic acid**. These ingredients function differently but achieve similar results — they accelerate the loss of dead skin cells to reduce pore blockage. You can spot treat acne with benzoyl peroxide.

Living with acne can be frustrating and stressful; however, you can take a proactive role in reducing the toll acne takes on your skin by educating yourself about home care. Talk to your dermatologist or skincare professional about products that are known to be effective and determine the best home remedy for you to use so you can move confidently toward an effective regimen.

## 4 Anti-Acne Power Foods to Add to Your Diet

If you suffer from regular acne breakouts, you know how frustrating and painful it can be. While there is no known cure for acne, there are treatments to keep your skin healthy and to help manage breakouts. One of the easiest ways to start is to simply incorporate four key anti-acne foods into your diet. They will help keep your skin looking its best. Incorporate these four anti-acne selections into your daily menu to keep your skin healthy and blemish-free.

**Omega-3 fatty acids** — According to the University of Maryland Medical Center, many clinicians are now recommending flaxseed, which is high in omega-3 fatty acids, as an acne treatment. Several studies have been conducted on the connection between fish oil and acne, and most of the results have been very favorable.

In addition to acting as an anti-acne agent, omega-3 fatty acids provide a host of other health benefits, particularly for the cardiovascular system. Common sources of omega-3s include:

❖ Fatty fish like salmon, tuna, mackerel and lake trout

❖ Nuts like walnuts, Brazil nuts and soy nuts

❖ Pumpkin seeds

❖ Flaxseeds and flaxseed oil

❖ Olive and soybean oil

**Berries**—Strawberries, blueberries, and raspberries all pack a powerful antioxidant punch. Antioxidants fight free radicals which damage cells, lead to signs of aging, and present a higher risk for disease. Antioxidants also provide a boost to the immune system, keeping the entire body healthier.

Since the skin is the largest organ of the body, it stands to reason that the health benefits of antioxidants positively affect the skin as well. And healthier skin means a complexion that is less prone to acne breakouts.

**Low-fat yogurt**—Yogurt is rich in probiotics, which promote the growth of good bacteria in the body. The root cause of acne breakouts is the bacteria known as p. acnes. Let the good bacteria in yogurt help you fight the bad bacteria.

Probiotics are only found in yogurt containing live cultures, so make sure the product you choose states that it contains live cultures. In addition to clearer skin, yogurt promotes a healthier immune system and a more efficient digestive system.

**Dark, leafy greens**—Popeye ate spinach to gain strength, but this popular green veggie is also an effective acne treatment. Dark, leafy greens like spinach, kale, and collard greens pack a potent level of vitamins and minerals that promote a healthier body overall. These vegetables are rich in the antioxidant nutrients that keep the skin supple, glowing, and acne-free.

**Zinc**—A common mineral found in greens, zink is another effective acne treatment because it regulates the production of sebum. An overabundance of sebum leads to acne breakouts, so reducing sebum production is an essential step in eliminating blemishes.

Eating right is the first step toward more beautiful, blemish-free skin. With these four anti-acne foods added to your daily diet, you skin will be clearer and you'll realize a host of other health benefits as well.

## ◈ TEEN ACNE

The angst of teen acne can be summed up in the following incident:

A teenager, getting ready to go out for the night, stops in front of the mirror for one last look before going out. All of a sudden she notices a huge zit on her nose and screams bloody murder. In a panic she cancels her plans for the night.

This is what acne does to most teens. Being a teenager is not easy. They have to deal with raging hormones, mood swings, all the irritations of puberty, and then, like the final straw, acne sets in. Nearly nine out of every eleven teens suffer from acne.

## What is Teen Acne?

Teen acne is known as acne vulgaris. It appears when the oil glands are overactive and become red, inflamed, or plugged. Acne appears on the skin in the form of bumps. Teen acne occurs typically because of the various hormonal changes occurring in the body during puberty, and it is usually most prolific on the face and the neck.

## The Four Common Forms of Teen Acne

1.  **Whiteheads:** Whiteheads are small white bumps on the skin. They appear when a pore is blocked and begins to bulge or swell under the skin.

2.  **Blackheads:** Blackheads are black bumps on the skin. They also appear when a pore gets blocked but in this case, the pore remains open allowing the top layer to turn black due to bacteria, sebum, dead skin cells, or dirt.

3.  **Nodules:** These are a more serious kind of acne. They are pimples which are red or swollen due to infection of the skin tissue around the area of the blocked pores. Nodules are hard to the touch, and are more painful than other types of acne.

4.  **Cysts:** Cysts are pus-filled pimples which may result in scarring.

## How to Take Care of Teen Acne

There are many steps that can be taken to fight teen acne, (e.g., eating right, using effective acne products, etc.). Teen acne is caused when the skin starts to excrete excess oil, so the best thing to do in this scenario is wash your face twice daily with an antibacterial soap, and eliminate oily food and snacks from your diet. So, the next time you experience a bout of teen acne, just make a few small changes to your everyday routine to keep it under control.

## ◈ ADULT ACNE

Teens aren't the only ones that battle acne. Adults are also subject to outbreaks. Adult acne may occur for a number of reasons: too much stress, inappropriate cosmetic products, hormone changes, and as a reaction to birth control pills. When you are under stress, the body starts to produce excess oil which can result in adult acne. If you use poor-quality cosmetic products, your pores may be affected by bacteria that lead to adult acne. However, the most common cause for adult acne is a fluctuation in hormone levels.

When this happens, the sebaceous glands in your skin may overact, making them ripe for an onset of acne. Adult acne usually starts with the appearance of blackheads. The thing to understand is that blackheads are not actually dirt; rather they are clogged pores that turn black. Blackheads can evolve into pimples if they get inflamed or infected. They can also turn into whiteheads or pustules, which are very painful and may result in scarring. Luckily, blackheads can easily be removed by scrubbing the face daily with a good quality scrub and blackhead removal strips. What separates adult acne from other types of acne is that it can be controlled through the use of various acne care products and regular, diligent care with scrubs, toners, and facials.

## 3 Powerful Ingredients that Get to the Root of Adult Acne

You may have thought you could say goodbye to blemishes and breakouts when you exited your teen years, but for many adults that is simply not the case. Acne can continue well into adulthood, perpetuating the embarrassment and pain of this skin condition.

The good news is that there are now effective ingredients that keep breakouts at bay while conditioning and toning your skin. Let's look at three key acne-fighting ingredients and a skin-care line that offers these three ingredients in its formulas:

1. **Glycolic acid** is an alpha hydroxy acid derived from sugar cane. It is perhaps best known as an exfoliating agent used in many skincare products, but it is particularly effective in formulas designed to treat adult acne.

   Glycolic acid works by penetrating the outer layers of the skin and sloughing off dead, dry cells, revealing the softer, smoother skin underneath. This ingredient is potent, so a little goes a long way. It works best when combined with soothing agents that replenish the moisture glycolic acid tends to strip away. Glycolic acid also makes skin more sensitive to the sun, so protection is recommended whenever you use skincare products containing glycolic acid.

2. **Salicylic acid** is another popular ingredient in adult acne skincare products. A beta hydroxyl acid, salicylic acid is particularly effective in treating whiteheads and blackheads. Like glycolic acid, salicylic acid penetrates follicles, getting underneath the outer layer of the skin to shed dead, dry skin cells that cause dull looking skin and spark breakouts. This substance may cause minor skin irritation initially, but reactions can be easily managed by using smaller amounts of the product until the skin becomes accustomed to it.

3. **Vitamin A** — While oral vitamin A has been used for years to treat adult acne, a topical version of the substance can be found in many acne skincare products. Usually labeled Retin A in formulas, this vitamin A derivative works by exfoliating the skin and is particularly effective in treating blackheads. Vitamin A/Retin A can cause redness and irritation when used in excess. It may also make skin more sensitive to UV rays, so sun protection is a must.

## The Triple Threat

While all of these ingredients are effective in treating adult acne, it is difficult to find a skincare line that offers all three in combination. MD Formulations is one of the few companies that provide a combination of these three ingredients in their acne skincare products.

**Alpha Beta Daily Peel** is just one of their excellent products. It uses a two-step process to address adult acne. The first step provides a hefty dose of glycolic acid and salicylic acid to effectively exfoliate skin and prevent future breakouts. The second step provides soothing vitamins, including vitamin A, to recondition skin — leaving it softer and smoother after treatment.

Treating adult acne isn't difficult as long as you use the right ingredients. With the three substances listed above in your skincare repertoire, you can keep breakouts at bay and enjoy softer, clearer skin.

## ❖ BODY ACNE

Acne is not limited to the face. In fact, body acne plagues a lot of people. Body acne can appear anywhere on the body — on the back, chest, arms and legs. Most people who suffer from facial acne also have some degree of body acne. Just as with facial breakouts, body acne occurs when the sebaceous glands in the body overact and produce too much sebum and oil. Body acne manifests in the same four basic forms as teen acne: blackheads, whiteheads, nodules/pustules, and cysts. Body acne worsens if the skin is irritated by damp clothing. You should wear fabrics that allow your skin to breathe (e.g. all-cotton) in order to avoid irritation to the skin and prevent back, chest, or body acne. If you perspire to the point that your clothes are damp, change into dry ones. Shower regularly, twice daily if necessary, and use an antibacterial soap or acne body wash. There are two basic treatments for body acne:

1.  Light cases can be cured by keeping the skin clean. After bathing, dry thoroughly and use a 10% alpha hydroxy acid to keep the skin clear and acne-free.

2.  In more severe cases, cleanse the skin thoroughly, and then apply small quantities of benzoyl peroxide and alpha hydroxyl acid.

Back and chest acne can be cured by following the steps just mentioned. Keep stress levels low, and bathe frequently, so that the skin on your body remains clean and any chance of body acne is completely eliminated.

## ◆ ACNE SCARS

## What Causes Acne Scars?

When acne becomes inflamed, forming pustules or cysts, the clogged pores swell with excess oils, dead skin cells, and bacteria that can fester. Swelling causes the wall of the follicle to break. When breakage occurs deep in the dermal layer, the skin tissue is destroyed and a scar forms over it. Scarring is the result of new collagen forming over damaged areas in an effort to fix the skin's tissues. However, this process of internal repair does not produce perfect results. If there is a loss of tissue, as is often the case, a crater will be left on the skin's surface.

## Social Effects of Acne Scarring

Most cases of severe acne occur among teenagers or young adults. The effects of acne can be socially and psychologically devastating. The scarring that often results is traumatic. Acne can lead to social inhibition, poor self-esteem, anxiety, and depression.

## Treatment Options

People do not have to live with acne scars forever. There are treatment options available. One such treatment is laser acne scar treatment. This is effective, but it is quite expensive. There are different types of lasers used:

❖ **Non-ablative lasers** are safe to use, and do not remove the epidermal layer of the skin.

❖ **Pulse dye lasers** remove the redness caused by acne scars.

❖ **Fractionated lasers** remodel scarred depressions.

Acne scar creams can be useful in treating scarring. A cream with cortisone can reduce inflammation and redness, and a cream that counteracts hyperpigmentation can be used on visible scars. Over-the-counter lightening creams may make scars look more natural, but they can do nothing to repair indentations.

Dermal fillers are another good treatment for scars. These fillers plump indented scars, similar to the way they fill in wrinkles. These fillers come in many forms, such as collagen, hyaluronic acid, fat cells, calcium hydroxylapatite, polymers, and microscopic plastic beads.

## ◈ ACNE PRODUCTS AND TREATMENTS REVIEWS

With so many products on the market, choosing a good acne product can be difficult; but when you're looking for the right ingredients and are armed with reliable product recommendations, it becomes a lot easier. We've been talking to consumers for years about their acne — asking which products helped, and which ones didn't. We've compiled a list to review some of the most popular acne products.

**B. Kamins** first developed a product to treat hormone-deprived skin using the trademarked technology *Bio-Maple Compound.*

Ben Kaminsky, a Canadian dermalogical chemist, derived the Bio-Maple Compound from purified sap from the Canadian Acer Saccharun Maple Trees. The Bio-Maple Compound is made up of complex physiological humectants, anti-oxidants, and penetrating moisturizers that contain mono and polysaccharides, amino peptides, and vegetable hormones. B. Kamins Bio-Maple Compound has been scientifically proven to maintain the skin's natural pH balance while protecting it from microorganisms that cause blemishes and irritations.

A chemist at B. Kamins first produced a Bio-Maple Compound clinical skincare product to treat menopausal women and women with hormone-deprived dry skin. The product used a nutrient replacement cream to help repair tissues. B. Kamins later discovered that hormonal changes were a contributing factor in adult acne and began to use the Bio-Maple Compound to produce acne skincare products.

B. Kamins has acne products for both adolescent and adult acne that are formulated to eliminate pimples and prevent breakouts using a combination of Bio-Maple Compound and salicylic acid. This powerful combination cleans the skin, controls bacteria, and reduces oils.

B. Kamins has six acne fighting products in their line: Corrective Mattifier, Matte Moisturizer, Purifying Masque, Hydrating Acne Wash, Blemish Gel, and Anti-Blemish Pads. It also produces an acne starter kit that contains one of each of the B. Kamins acne fighting products.

B. Kamins products were specifically designed to treat both normal and problematic skin (e.g., rosaceous, acne-prone, sun-damaged, hormone-deprived mature skin, and sensitive skin) and have proven to be effective in reducing acne breakouts.

**BioElements** has developed a revolutionary skincare system to control acne and keep skin healthy and clean. BioElements Skincare uses the Biotype System to customize formulas for different skin types and conditions. BioElements uses a blend of salicylic acid and natural vitamins and minerals to thoroughly clean the skin and remove dirt, oils, and bacteria without stripping the skin and making it dry. BioElements has developed a four-part cleaning system that provides 24-hour protection against acne. The BioElements Acne Prevention Cleaning System contains BioElements Spotless Cleanser, BioElements Active Astringent, BioElements Amino Mask, and BioElements Acne Plex.

The BioElements acne product line contains salicylic acid, a powerful and effective ingredient used to prevent acne breakouts. BioElements products use deep cleansing, exfoliation, and a custom blend of salicylic acid serums to aid in the prevention of acne breakouts. Pineapple, papaya, and witch hazel are also used in the products as powerful, all-natural cleaning agents.

BioElements skincare products won't cause clogged pores (which can result in blemishes). BioElements acne prevention skincare products focus on preventing clogged pores while removing excess oils and leaving the skin healthy with a matte, non-oily finish.

Skincare is only effective if you use the right formulations and regimen. BioElements Skincare has produced complete skincare systems to assist people in their regimen to effectively maintain healthy, acne-free skin. BioElements Skincare is a professional skincare line used by specialists and consumers worldwide.

**BioMedic by La Roche Posay** is a leader in skincare technology. It offers a complete professional line of products for in-office corrective procedures of the skin. La Roche Posay, located in Paris, uses thermal spring water in its products. These products also have a high concentration of selenium—an anti-inflammatory that effectively softens and soothes irritated skin following in-office spa treatments—which has a long history of producing successful skincare benefits.

La Roche Posay skincare products can be found in skincare clinics around the world, and are widely recommended by the dermatologist community. Its skincare products are extremely effective in healing skin irritations, acne breakouts, and skin sensitivities because all of their products are hypoallergenic, paraben-free, and fragrance-free.

La Roche Posay Effaclar products are recommended for acne-prone and problematic skin types. The Effaclar Deep Cleaning Foaming Cream and Purifying Foaming Gel are daily cleansers that remove excess oils and tighten pores without drying the skin. When these products are coupled with the Effaclar Toner, a micro-exfoliate that unclogs pores, your skin will feel refreshed and clean.

La Roche Posay Effaclar also produces an Intensive Acne Spot Treatment that combines salicylic acid and benzoyl peroxide to combat individual blemishes. Effaclar Acne Treatment Fluid and Moisturizers are acne-fighting products that are part of the La Roche Posay Effaclar acne treatment product line.

La Roche Posay Effaclar products will keep skin clean, fresh, and acne-free. The company continues to produce scientifically proven products for both office and home use. They are appropriate for the advanced treatment of all types of skin conditions.

**Celazome** is produced by the Florida cosmaceuticals company Dermazone. Dermazone produces scientific products that meet specific skincare needs for all skin types and conditions. Celazome skincare products are produced with a patented delivery system called Lyphazome. Lyphazomes are natural nanospheres, 1/50th the size of regular skin cells, that penetrate the epidermis and effectively deliver ingredients deep below the skin's surface. Celazome products are used worldwide by professional skincare practitioners and in skincare clinics.

Celazome produces a collection of skincare products designed to target specific skin conditions using the Lyphazome natural nanospheres. Celazome's products are pharmaceutical strength and use a blend of natural bioactives to treat and repair the skin while providing acne control, wrinkle reduction, and anti-aging properties. They also carry daily skincare products.

Celazome designed a skincare system specifically for acne control and prevention. The Celazome O-PLEX system cleans the skin and prevents new blemishes from forming by using its deep-cleaning, trademarked Complex Origanum.

The Celazome O-Plex system is a three-part skincare system for acne control. The three products in the Celazome O-Plex system are O-Plex Wash, O-Plex Mist, and O-Plex Control. Celazome O-Plex Wash removes excess oils and bacteria. O-Plex Mist tightens pores and maintains oil control. O-Plex Control treats acne and prevents future breakouts. The Celazome O-Plex system is a powerful skincare regimen for the treatment of acne. Celazome O-Plex also produces O-Plex Target with Lyphazome technology cream that specifically targets blemishes using a sulphur, tea tree oil, and Origanium complex. O-Plex Target eliminates blemishes and prevents future breakouts.

**Clean Start By Dermalogica** is a complete skincare system specifically designed for teens to promote healthy skin and help control acne. Dermalogica is a skincare company that has been producing skincare products for over 25 years. The founder, Jane Wurwand, saw a need for teen skincare and developed the Clean Start products.

The Clean Start product line is affordable and helps teens maintain skin health through the use of natural ingredients that are gentle and won't damage the skin. Clean Start promotes its products through skincare education and programs that teens find interesting; Clean Start even invited a group of teens to participate in developing the line by having them work with the company on the package and label designs.

Teen acne can be controlled through proper skincare, and Clean Start products help teens achieve healthy looking, acne-free skin. The Clean Start acne control cleansing product line consists of eight products that provide dual-action cleansing to balance the skin, leaving it clean and oil-free. Clean Start products are non-clogging and help keep pores clear of dirt and oils that cause blemishes.

Clean Start All Over Clear is a foaming wash that can be used in the shower. It is suitable for the face, back, and chest. Clean Start All Over Clear is a favorite with teens. It is dispensed as a light mist that can be used to control shine and prevent acne breakouts. The light mist cools and refreshes the skin on contact. It contains sesame seed, licorice, burdock, and argan extracts that control oils and hydrate the skin while protecting it from environmental elements.

Clean Start also produces a set of cleansers, masks, acne spot treatments, and moisturizers for the face and lips. The Clean Start product line is effective in controlling teen acne and preventing blemish breakouts.

**Dermanew Products** and the **Dermanew Microdermabrasion System** were founded by Amby Longhofer and her husband Dean Rhodes. Dermanew products offer revolutionary treatments for all skin types and conditions.

The Dermanew home microdermabrasion products were modeled after the professional microdermabrasion spa treatments offered at salons throughout the world. Dermanew saw a need for a home version of microdermabrasion for clients that couldn't afford continuous salon treatments. These products are designed for anti-aging, acne, and problematic skin that require deep cleansing through microdermabrasion. The Dermanew Microdermabrasion System is easy to use and the results can be seen after just one treatment. The handheld skin resurfacer used with the Dermanew Acne and Oil Clarifying Cream provide deep cleansing for pores, remove dirt, oils, and bacteria, and leave skin polished and refreshed. The deep cleansing properties of the Acne and Oil Clarifying Cream help prevent future blemish breakouts through the use of salicylic acid and natural extracts.

Dermanew has daily-use acne controlling products to help maintain the skin's overall health before and after microdermabrasion treatments. The Dermanew Decongestive Cleanser is a deep cleaning gel ideal for pre-cleaning the skin prior to microdermabrasion. It can also be used daily to keep the skin clean and fresh.

The Dermanew Acne Active Hydrator is an oil-free moisturizer that maintains hydration without clogging pores even as it protects the skin from environmental factors. The Dermanew Toning Agent is a powerful astringent that actively reduces oil and bacteria following cleansing.

The Dermanew Microdermabrasion Acne and Oil Control System and the Dermanew daily skincare treatment products are guaranteed to control acne and prevent breakouts. They are designed for adolescents and adults, and offer professional strength acne-controlling products for home use.

**GloProfessional** is the manufacturer of GloMineral Make Up and the GloTherapeutics Skincare Collection. GloProfessional has created a complete line of skincare products and makeup for all skin types and conditions. GloMineral makeup offers a collection of camouflaging concealers and foundation products that completely hide skin imperfections and discolorations without clogging pores. GloMineral is an all-natural makeup using a three-part system (GloCamofluage, GloPressed Base, and GloConcealer) to completely transform the look of the skin.

GloTherapeutics are clinically proven products developed to clean, refresh, and treat skin conditions, and are known to be some of the best acne products on the market today. GloTherapeutics has a complete line for acne control and problematic skin. GloTherapeutics GloClear Acne Cleanser is excellent for treating acne and preventing future breakouts.

GloTherapeutics GloClear Acne Cleanser contains salicylic acid, scrubbing bubbles, and apple enzymes that thoroughly wash away bacteria, excess oil, and dirt, leaving skin soft, smooth, and clean.

GloTherapeutics Clear Complexion Pads provide an effective way to remove acne-causing bacteria and balance the skin's natural pH through the use of salicylic acid, citric acid, and spearmint. It has also produced a full line of products that clean, protect, and moisturize acne and oil-prone skin.

**Glytone Skincare** products were created by pharmacists who initially developed physician-only glycolic acid products for professional skincare clinics. Later its products became available for home use under the guidance of professional skincare specialists.

Glytone Skincare products have nine distinctive skincare systems designed for specific skin types and conditions. They are:

❖ Professional

❖ Step up

❖ Post op

❖ Antioxidant

❖ Clarifying

❖ Acne

❖ Essentials

❖ Body

❖ Sun care

The Glytone Acne home skincare system is designed to prevent the recurrence of acne breakouts and helps keep skin healthy, clean, and clear. Glytone acne-fighting formulas contain cleaners, toners, masks, lotions, and sprays. Glytone even introduced an Acne Treatment Kit containing the main skincare products to give its clients a comprehensive, one-package start for their at home skincare regimen.

Glytone's Acne Facial Cleanser and Cleansing Toner contain salicylic acid, a powerful acne-fighting ingredient that removes dead skin cells and reduces acne-producing bacteria. Its Exfoliating Gel Wash is a deep cleansing skincare treatment that contains glycolic acid. Other developments include the Benzoyl Peroxide Acne Gel for periodic breakouts and the Acne Facial Masque for spa-like deep cleansing facial treatments.

A unique product in the Glytone Acne prevention skincare line is Glytone Back Acne Spray with salicylic acid. The spray dries quickly, and the unique pump is designed to work even when held upside down for easy application. Clients with back acne will get both relief and acne control from Glytone Back Acne Spray.

**Jurlique Skincare** offers all-natural skincare products for the entire body made from a blend of herbs and rich botanicals. Many of the plant extracts and flowers found in Jurlique products are grown on the company farm in South Australia.

Jurlique Skincare products are used to treat all skin types and conditions. Its signature product is Rosewater Balancing Mist, which uses 8000 rose petals to extract the rose oil found in every bottle. Rose oil is used as the base for many of the Jurlique skincare products.

Jurlique Skincare products contain powerful antidotes for acne. Jurlique Blemish Cream is an all-natural, oil-balancing cream that helps clean acne-prone skin with Calendula, witch hazel, and tea tree oil. Jurlique's Purifying Mask is a rich clay cream made of herbal extracts that removes dead skin cells, excessive oils, and dirt leaving behind a clear, balanced skin tone. Jurlique Skincare products use only naturally grown ingredients in their skincare products, with none of the harsh chemicals or ingredients normally used in acne-fighting skincare products.

Jurlique produces a line of herbal recovery formulas and essential oils. Many people find relief from acne with the antimicrobial Tea Tree Essential Oil used in a vaporizer or burner. The company's Calendula Lotion, used for many skin types including acne-prone skin, is an herbal blend that improves the overall health of the skin and restores its natural balance.

Jurlique Skincare continues to develop products using homegrown natural botanicals to produce advanced skincare. Jurlique Skincare products used daily keep skin clean and oil-free, reduce the risk of outbreaks, and keep skin healthy-looking.

**MD Formulations** is a leader in skincare technology using a patented glycolic compound in their skincare products. Glycolic acid has many benefits for the skin, but it can be very damaging and irritating if the skin is sensitive. MD Formulations Glycolic Compound uses glycolic acid in a non-irritating formula so it is suitable for sensitive and problematic skin types. MD Formulations Glycolic Compound offers the benefits of glycolic acid without causing sensitivity or irritation.

MD Formulations developed a skincare treatment kit specifically designed to control adult acne breakouts and to keep skin clean and clear of blemishes.

The MD Formulations Adult Anti-Blemish Kit contains the following five acne-controlling products:

❖ Facial Cleanser

❖ Continuous Renewal Serum

❖ Vit-A-Plus Clearing Complex

❖ Moisturize Defense Antioxidant Lotion

❖ Total Protector 30

The kit, when used daily, can significantly improve the overall health of the skin while controlling future acne breakouts.

The MD Formulations Vit-A-Plus Body Clearing Complex Spray is a combination of BHA, AHA, and retinol-pure vitamin A that helps clean out pores and control blemish breakouts. It contains rosemary, salicylic acid, and lactic acid—all working together to exfoliate, smooth, and relax the skin.

**Neostrata** is a U.S skincare company known worldwide. It has developed some of the most popular doctor-recommended skincare brands, including NeoStrata, Coverblend, NeoCeuticals, NeoStrata Therapeutics, and the Exuviance brand.

NeoStrata products are physician-dispensed for advanced skincare. Neostrata has developed skincare solutions for numerous conditions, including rosacea, sensitive skin, oily skin, acne-prone skin, keratosis pilaris, psorasis, dry skin, and eczema. Neostrata produces a full range of acne control skincare products in its NeoStrata and NeoCeuticals lines. The line employs the patented NeoHydroxy Complex which penetrates deep into the skin to unclog pores and eliminate blemishes and is popular for its soap-free cleansers. The NeoStrata Antibacterial Facial Cleanser is a soap-free cleanser that contains triclosan, pro-vitamin B5, and chamomile extract which act together to thoroughly clean the skin, remove excess oils, and reduce the bacteria that cause acne. Neoceuticals Antibacterial Facial Cleanser contains 2% salicylic acid, which helps to clear blemishes and prevent new acne without drying the skin

NeoStrata has a complete skincare regimen for acne-troubled skin. NeoStrata Oily Skin Solution, Renewal Cream, and Oil Free Lotion with SPF 15 are all part of the NeoStrata acne and oily skincare collection. Using this collection daily can significantly reduce breakouts and keep oil under control, leaving your skin looking healthy and clear while feeling smooth and soft.

**PCA Skin** was founded in 1991 by Margaret Ancira, a licensed aesthetician, who collaborated with physicians and scientists to develop a skincare line that used scientifically researched ingredients to treat many common skin conditions.

PCA Skin is a leading innovator in the professional skincare industry and was one of the first companies to develop a chemical peel formulation for professional skin treatments. PCA Skin has developed a wide range of potent skincare products for home use that would normally be found only in professional skincare clinics. Its products are designed for all types of skin and skin conditions, but its primary focus is on anti-aging and acne-control.

PCA Skin developed a full line of professional acne treatment products to help control the oil that leads to clogged pores, resulting in blackheads and pimples. PCA Skin pHaze 31 BPO 5% Cleanser and pHaze Acne Gel both contain benzoyl peroxide, a scientifically proven ingredient that removes acne-causing bacteria on the skin, thereby helping to control breakouts. The PCA Skin pHaze 32 Blemish Control Bar is an antibacterial cleansing agent that also aids in reducing bacteria on the skin's surface. PCA Skin pHaze 33 Acne Cream is a topical acne solution made from 5% liquid benzoyl peroxide.

**Peter Thomas Roth** was founded in 1993 when Peter Roth began developing skincare products in the old Hungarian skin healing tradition. Over the years, Peter Thomas Roth has developed over 100 products, now available worldwide through skincare clinics and spas. Peter Thomas Roth skin-care products are designed to treat various conditions on the face, hands, body, and scalp; they are suitable for all types of skin. Peter Thomas Roth products include skincare solutions for acne-control, anti-aging, skin brightening, oil control, cleansing, moisturizing oil control, and sun protection.

Peter Thomas Roth acne solution products were designed for both adolescents and adults to address the underlying, contributing factors that cause acne breakouts. Its acne products reduce excessive oil, eliminate the bacteria that cause acne to form, remove dead skin cells, and include all-day oil control lotions, Beta Hydroxy Acne fighting cleansers, blemish buffing (bead) face and body wash, acne spot treatments, and cooling masques.

The Peter Thomas Roth line of products has won many skincare and health industry awards. In 2009 the award for Best Peel Product was awarded to Peter Thomas Roth by Allure Magazine for its Gentle Complexion Correction Pads—cleansing pads that clean pores and prevent blackheads.

Peter Thomas Roth has also developed a skincare line specifically for men that offers face, hair, and body cleansers, shaving cream, and aftershave gel that keeps men's skin healthy and blemish-free. Peter Thomas Roth has a wide selection of products for every type of skin for both genders. All Peter Thomas Roth products have been clinically tested for their effectiveness.

**Pevonia Botanica Skincare** (acne treatment) offers professional spa products worldwide through exclusive luxury spas and skincare clinics. Pevonia Botanica Skincare Company is located in Daytona Beach, Florida, and has been producing award-winning skincare products since 1991.

Pevonia Botanica Skincare produces 100% natural skincare products for all types of skin conditions and treatments. This company provides the leading professional spa treatments for acne and problematic skin and offers one of the top-selling acne product lines for home maintenance.

Pevonia Botanica Skincare's home acne treatment products are made from all-natural organic extracts similar to those found in leading Pevonia Spas. They keep skin clean and free from acne-causing bacteria. Pevonia developed a full line of teenage acne treatments using organic benzoyl peroxide and salicylic acid for home use. These daily cleansing products control oil and prevent acne breakouts. The Pevonia SpaTeen blemish control product line includes the SpaTeen Blemished Skin Mask, Blemished Skin Cleanser, Blemished Skin Toner, Blemished Moisturizer, and Blemish-B-Gone Spot Treatment.

Its products for adults clean, heal, and moisturize acne and problematic skin without clogging pores. They also prevent breakouts without harsh chemicals or alcohol.

The Pevonia Acne Treatment line for home use includes Clarigel, Problematic Skin Lotion, Problematic Skincare Cream, a Purifying Skin Mask, and a Blemish Spot Treatment. These products are very effective in preventing and controlling acne, and can be used by both men and women to maintain youthful, healthy, and acne-free skin.

**Phytomer Skincare** products are marine-based cosmetology solutions known throughout the world. Phytomer Skincare is based in Saint Malo and has been developing all-natural skincare products for more than 35 years. These products draw on the natural ingredient phytomer found in ocean plants and algae. Phytomer Skincare uses a scientific process in order to obtain *oigomer*, a seawater concentrate proven to hydrate and improve skin health.

Phytomer Skincare offers a full range of products that address everything from cleansing and toning, to anti-aging prevention, to acne control. Phytomer Oligopur Purifying Cleansing Gel contains natural antibacterial seaweed extract that gently removes excess oils and thoroughly cleanses the skin to prevent acne breakouts without over-drying. The Phytomer Oligopur Purifying AcniControl fluid for problem skin uses natural marine extracts to control oil, reduce inflammation, and balance the skin.

Acne prevention begins with a proper skincare regimen, regular daily cleansing, oil control, protection, and moisturizing. The Phytomer cleansing and toning treatments are made from Seagorse, sorenia aromatic marine water that leaves skin clean and soft. The Oligo Pur Line cleans and purifies the skin with high-performance moisturizers that contain pheohydrane, a brown algae that softens and protects the skin. Phytomer produces an anti-pollution complex called Soufflé Marine Breeze Energizing Oxygenating Serum. It is made with marine flowers to protect the skin from adverse environmental conditions. The Oxygenating Serum is developed from a combination of coastal plants, armeria maritime, and sea sugar.

**SkinMedica** was developed by Dr. Richard Fitzpatrick who believed that the skin was self-healing. SkinMedica uses advanced skincare ingredients such as vitamin C, vitamin E, retinol and TNS (a patented blend of growth factors, soluble collagen, antioxidants, and matrix proteins) to boost the skin's natural ability to heal itself.

SkinMedica developed a complete acne skincare system using therapeutic antiseptics to provide deep pore cleaning while removing dirt, oils, and acne-forming bacteria and to help prevent future breakouts. The SkinMedica Acne Skincare System contains a purifying foaming wash, a purifying toner, and an acne treatment lotion. The SkinMedica Purifying Foaming Wash and Purifying Toner contain 2% salicylic acid to unclog pores and remove dead skin cells. SkinMedica Acne Treatment Lotion contains 2.5% benzoyl peroxide, willow bark extract (a natural source of salicylic acid), witch hazel (a natural healing and anti-inflammatory ingredient), Salvia Officinalis (Sage) and Leaf Extract (an antibacterial and anti-inflammatory ingredient). Together, the SkinMedica Acne Treatment Lotion ingredients eliminate acne-forming bacteria and reduce inflammation, leaving clean, clear skin behind. All the products in the SkinMedica Skincare System were developed to work together as a daily skincare regimen that controls acne and maintains healthy, clear skin without dehydration or irritation.

SkinMedica is committed to the research and development of new skincare products to combat aging and acne-prone skin. SkinMedica is known globally, and has been recognized on many national television shows such as Dr. Oz, Good Morning America, and the Doctors for its beneficial skincare treatments.

**Sothys Paris Professional Skincare Company** opened in France in 1946. It was acquired by the Mas Family (the current owners) in 1966. Sothys Paris has been developing professional skincare products for more than 60 years. Today its skincare products are sold worldwide and the company is a leader in the skincare industry. Its products are promoted through luxury spas and salons.

Sothys Paris uses marine and botanical extracts along with certified, active organic ingredients to produce effective, professional cosmaceuticals for advanced skincare therapies. Sothys produces skincare products for acne control, anti-aging, de-stressing, eye contouring, lip smoothing, and hand and body treatments.

The Correcting Treatment collection includes a Hydra-Matt Fluid, Active Cream, and Purifying Serum. The Sothys Paris Hydra-Matt Fluid is a light gel used to protect and moisturize the skin. Sothys Paris Active Cream uses liquorice extract and biostimuline from sweet corn to provide a soothing and soft lotion for the skin. Sothys Paris' Purifying Serum is applied directly to blemishes to reduce inflammation and cleanse the inflamed area. Using the Sothys Paris Professional Correcting Treatment line of products as a daily skincare regimen keeps skin clean and blemish free while making it healthier and softer.

**Vivier Pharma** is a Canadian company located in Montreal, Quebec. It was founded in 1997 by Jess Vivier. Vivier Pharma manufactures VivierSkin, SkinTx, and Lidomax specialty products for skincare specialists and dermatologists worldwide. The SkinTx Skin Treatment System was specifically designed to help restore and correct or improve irregular skin conditions such as hyperpigmentation, aging, skin texture, and acne prone skin. SkinTx uses a combination of Retinol, Hydroquinone, alpha hydroxy acids, and vitamin C to repair and restore skin to a healthier condition.

SkinTx offers professional strength products that are gentle but extremely effective in cleaning the skin and removing excess oils and dirt. It unclogs pores and balances the skin's natural pH. SkinTx cleansers are available in a gentle cleansing form, a foaming gel, micro scrub gel, and a micro scrub cream formula designed specifically for different skin types and cleansing needs. SkinTx also offers a toner and a deep cleansing astringent. All SkinTx Products are designed to thoroughly clean the skin by removing environmental impurities and acne forming bacteria.

Vivier Pharma produced a SkinTx Starter System that includes all the necessary products to begin a daily, acne-fighting skin regimen. The SkinTx Starter System Program for acne consists of 8 full-size products:

❖ Foaming gel

❖ Astringent

❖ Clarite 4

❖ Exfoliant Forte

❖ Active 4

❖ Retinol SR Facial Treatment

❖ Physical Facial Block SPF 30

❖ Eye cream

These products were chosen for their effectiveness in caring for acne prone skin. Using the SkinTx Starter System helps control oil, inflammation, and acne breakouts. Clients using the SkinTx Starter System Program also find that the products are effective in reducing blackheads and whiteheads. A daily regimen of SkinTx professional strength products help reduce blemish outbreaks and control acne, leaving skin feeling soft and looking healthy.

## ≈ 6 ∾

# SKIN CONDITIONS AND HOW TO FIGHT THEM

W anting beautiful skin and to look like all your favorite idols and movie stars is perfectly normal, but it can be devastating to have a skin condition that makes you question your own beauty. Unfortunately, this happens all too often, especially with teens who can believe that they are in competition with peers that have flawless skin. Teen usually want to fit in, but skin conditions, regardless of the source or severity, can definitely make a teen look and, more importantly, feel different.

If you have blemishes, itchy or blotchy red skin or cracked scaly skin, you may feel embarrassed and want to hide until it all goes away. Symptoms vary from one skin condition to another, but some of the more common are acne, psoriasis, and Rosacea.

Eczema is yet another skin condition that affects not only the face, but the hands and feet as well. Hyperpigmentation or melasma is another condition in which the skin is darker in some areas than on others, giving the skin a mottled or blotchy look.

## ◈ ECZEMA

Eczema or atopic dermatitis often starts in childhood but unfortunately it can follow you into adolescence and adulthood. It seems to run in families that are also subject to asthma or hay fever and other allergies. It is actually unclear what causes eczema, but it is believed to be a breakdown of the body's immune system. It is associated with dry skin that irritates and inflames. It flares up and then subsides at irregular intervals.

## What are the Symptoms of Eczema?

Typical symptoms of eczema include cracked and scaly skin that becomes thick and may exhibit small raised bumps. It is accompanied by severe itching that usually occurs at night and may cause the skin to crust over from repeated scratching. The skin gets red or gray-brown in patches and can be very sensitive and/or raw from the constant itching and scratching cycle.

Eczema can appear anywhere on the body, but is most often found on the feet, hands, elbows, knees and ankles. It can also show up on the face, neck and upper chest, and is especially debilitating when it occurs around the eyelids as scratching will not only cause redness but also swelling. Eyebrows and eyelashes are sometimes affected and you may notice an accompanying loss of hair with excessive scratching and rubbing in these sensitive areas.

## Other Things that Affect Eczema

Stress is a major factor in adverse changes that affect the body and it can definitely exacerbate existing eczema. Other conditions that can affect eczema include dry skin, rapid changes in temperature, cigarette smoke, perspiration, and long, hot showers or baths.

Some cleaners, soaps, or detergents can irritate the skin and cause your eczema to get worse. Foods like milk, fish, eggs, soy, or wheat are known to agitate this skin condition as will coarse clothing such as wool. Colds or other respiratory infections can cause eczema to reoccur.

# Finding Relief from Eczema

If you or a member of your family experiences the symptoms associated with eczema, and they do not abate within a few days, seek advice from a physician. Eczema is not curable, but it can be contained. There are treatments that will provide relief from the itching, but if left unattended, the itching may lead to infection.

Eczema makes the skin extremely dry so the goal is keep the skin moisturized with creams and lotions that are specifically formulated to treat the condition. These should be applied when the skin is damp—right after bathing or showering. Cold compresses may provide some relief. There are over the counter products that contain hydrocortisone that offer relief in mild cases, but people with more severe cases need to see a doctor to get a prescription for something stronger. He/she may also prescribe an antibiotic if there is an infection present. Antihistamines have been used successfully to reduce itching, and some people respond well to photo therapy that applies ultraviolet light to affected areas.

# How to Prevent Eczema Flare Ups

Many of the preventive measures used to prevent eczema flare ups are just common sense:

❖ Keep the skin moisturized and hydrated all the time.

❖ Avoid detergents, solvents, soaps, and other harsh products that might affect your skin.

❖ Avoid coarse fabrics like wool or other rough materials.

❖ Try not to become overheated.

❖ Minimize activities that cause excessive perspiration.

❖ Avoid strenuous activity in the heat.

❖ Stay away from environmental stressors like pollen, mold or animal dander.

❖ Reduce stress — this isn't easy in today's hectic world, but if you can avoid stressful situations you may be able to reduce the flare ups from eczema.

## ◈ Guard Against Skin Cancer

Over a million people in the United State are diagnosed with skin cancer each year. It is the most common form of cancer and can be one of the deadliest. Skin cancer is divided into three types:

❖ Basal cell carcinoma

❖ Squamous cell carcinoma

❖ Melanoma

Most people have the basal or squamous cell form that generally won't spread to other parts of the body, but it can develop into a malignant melanoma if not treated early. Melanoma is most common in people in their late twenties.

Skin cancer cases are increasing at an alarming rate, especially in fair-skinned people. People with light colored hair and blue or green eyes are at the greatest risk. People that freckle or sunburn easily may also be prime candidates for skin cancer. Other things that might affect a person's vulnerability are the presence of a large number of moles or a close family member with a history of skin cancer.

## Causes of Skin Cancer

The most common cause of skin cancer is excessive exposure to ultraviolet or UVA and UVB sun rays. Unfortunately, many Baby Boomers grew up without knowing how harmful the sun's rays could be to our skin. We soaked up the rays trying to achieve the ultimate tan, thinking that it made us look healthier. In fact, the exact opposite was true — sun rays have proved to be the cause of many skin cancers today.

The artificial light you're exposed to in tanning booths is another source of skin cancer. Younger people think the tanning booth is a healthy alternative to sun bathing, but they may be equally harmful to our skin. Exposure to tanning booths should be limited as with sun exposure. Skin cancer can also be caused by contact with chemicals like arsenic. Occupations like mining and farming that use these chemicals may put practitioners at risk. Other things that put us at risk for skin cancer are the hydrocarbons found in tar, oil, and soot, over-exposure to x-rays, and medications that impair the immune system.

## Symptoms of Skin Cancer

❖ **Basal cell carcinoma** appears as a small bump on the skin with blood vessels visible inside. It will develop a crust and bleed, acting like a sore that will not heal.

❖ **Squamous cell carcinoma** appears as a red, scaly, thickened patch of skin that may bleed and ulcerate. It can spread to healthy skin if not treated early.

❖ **Melanomas** are the malignant skin cancers that normally look like black or brown lesions on the skin. They may manifest as a change in the shape, color and/or size of a mole, or as a new patch of skin that is sore and might itch, ulcerate, or bleed. Often the sides of the lesion have irregular borders and are not symmetrical. Melanomas can be a mixture of several colors including: black, brown, tan, red, blue, or white. Any type of mole or suspicious-looking patches of skin that begin to change or increase in size should be immediately checked by a dermatologist.

## Treatment of Skin Cancer and Preventive Measures

If you develop skin cancer, a dermatologist will probably take a sample or biopsy of the affected skin area so that it can be examined to determine the extent of the disease. If you have basal or squamous cell carcinoma, these lesions can usually be removed surgically or through alternative treatments.

Malignant melanoma will probably require more extensive surgery and could require radiation or chemotherapy once the extent of the skin cancer is determined. In melanoma cases, an oncologist is often consulted as well.

Preventive measures include minimizing exposure to the sun's harmful UV rays by using a broad spectrum SPF protective sunscreen with a rating of 30 or more. Protective clothing such as wide brimmed hats and long sleeves are suggested when at the beach or pool to minimize excessive exposure to the sun's harmful rays. Keeping the skin well hydrated and moisturized as well as protected will keep it healthier and will hopefully deter any skin cancers from appearing.

## ◈ PROTECT YOUR SKIN FROM THE SUN AND MELASMA

Melasma is commonly found in women in their reproductive years, between 20 and 50 years of age. It usually occurs during pregnancy in women with olive or dark skin, and most typically in women of Hispanic, Asian, or Middle Eastern descent, but it can occur in anyone. It presents as a discoloration or hyperpigmentation of the skin that is brown, blue, gray, or tan. Occurrences seem to be related to excessive exposure to the sun, the use of birth control pills, and internal hormonal changes that occur during pregnancy.

Although melasma can be unattractive, it is a benign skin condition unrelated to any medical disorder and is considered relatively harmless. It is a skin condition that usually occurs only when a woman is pregnant, but it occasionally affects non-pregnant women for a few years and then goes away completely. Even though it is not considered serious, there is treatment available if needed.

### Factors that Influence Melasma

The exact cause of melasma is unknown, but it seems to be influenced by hormone replacement therapy, birth control pills and other medications such as anti-seizure medicines, race, and heredity. Exposure to sunlight especially without any protection or sunscreen is thought to be the leading cause of melasma with occurrences most often developing during the summer months when the sun is at its hottest and most intense.

Other factors that can influence melasma are endocrine dysfunction, nutritional deficiency, or hepatic dysfunction. The majority of cases occur during pregnancy (especially if there is a deficiency of folic acid) or with the use of oral contraceptives. Melasma can occur during menopause or if there are ovarian disorders that result in a hormone imbalance. Some deodorant soaps, toiletries, and scented cosmetics have been known to cause outbreaks of melasma.

## What Does Melasma Look Like?

Melasma primarily appears on the face as patches of brown discoloration or hyperpigmentation. It can occur on the cheeks, forehead, nose, chin, upper lip, and jaw. It can also appear on the arms, but these cases are rare. These dark patches skin are irregular in shape with uneven but symmetrical distribution on the sides of the nose, forehead, or cheeks.

## How Do You Treat Melasma?

You can keep melasma at bay and avoid outbreaks by using a sunscreen with a broad spectrum for UVA and UVB protection—one with an SPF rating of at least 30. Sunscreens should be used daily and exposure to the sun for long periods of time should be avoided. Discontinue the use of any cleansers, makeup, or other skin care products that irritate your skin.

Bleaching cream with hydroquinone is often used in the treatment of melasma to lighten the skin's hyperpigmentation and even out the skin tones; it should not be used during pregnancy, however. Laser treatments, chemical peels, or microdermabrasion are all treatments that can be used to treat melasma. Retin-A creams can be used at night to treat the areas of hyperpigmented skin.

## Other Methods of Prevention and Treatment

Antioxidant supplements can enhance the results of other melasma treatments. Natural lightening creams that contain antioxidants are also effective. Cleansers and mild soaps designed specifically for melasma minimize irritation. Calamine and other moisturizing lotions that contain nutrients and soothing extracts are great to keep the skin hydrated.

Excessive exposure to the sun seems to be the major trigger for melasma, so it is important that you use a sunscreen along with protective clothing if your skin is predisposed to melasma. Wide hats help as melasma occurs most frequently on the face. Protective facial makeup is also available to help keep skin tones even.

### ❖ HEALTHIER SKIN FOR PEOPLE WITH PSORIASIS

Psoriasis is a common chronic skin condition that affects people of all ages, although it is most common in young adults. It is a non-curable condition that can be embarrassing and cause emotional distress because of its unattractive appearance on the skin. It is often worse in cold weather and may come and go for no apparent reason throughout your life. It affects all races around the world, and all ages from small children to senior citizens. Caucasians are twice as susceptible to the disease as African Americans.

## What is Psoriasis?

While there is no known cause, psoriasis is assumed to be a combination of environmental and genetic factors that cause rapid skin cell reproduction which results in dry, red patches of thickened skin that develops into scales and flakes. It is usually found on the scalp, knees and elbows. Severe cases can cover a person's entire body.

## What are the Symptoms of Psoriasis?

Psoriasis not look the same everywhere on the body, but it often appears as small, flattened bumps on raised red or pink patches of skin. Because it is dry, it is also very flaky, but don't try to pull the flaky patches off as it may cause bleeding.

Several types of psoriasis look like small drops or liquid-filled blisters. These are usually found under the arms or in the navel or buttocks. There are also genital lesions that can be found on the penis. White spots on the fingernails might be nail psoriasis and psoriasis on the scalp often looks like dandruff.

## How Do You Treat Psoriasis?

Like most other skin conditions, the treatment of psoriasis depends on the severity of the condition. Mild cases that involve less than 10% of the body can be effectively treated with topical skin creams or lotions. Sometimes a local injection of steroids can help in particularly resistant areas.

Topical products are less effective on moderate psoriasis covering larger areas. This includes more severe cases as well because sometimes the very location of the outbreak may make it difficult to apply lotions or creams. Treatments for these more severe cases may include injections, pills, light treatments, or stronger medications with the treatment decision being based on the severity of the psoriasis. These stronger medications, however, may mean an increased risk for some people.

A common practice in psoriasis treatment is to rotate the treatments used every six to twelve months in order to minimize any possible side effects. An example might be to use light therapy for a year, and then switch to injections of biologic drugs to ensure that the individual is getting optimal treatments with minimum risks.

## How to Have Healthier Skin with Psoriasis

Psoriasis can develop spontaneously in people and then disappear just as suddenly. This chronic inflammatory skin condition can improve with proper care and may even go into remission. With so many types of treatments available, including light therapy and biologic drugs that offer promising results, psoriasis is definitely treatable and can be controlled.

If you have psoriasis, it is essential that you seek advice from a dermatologist or skin care professional. The skin care products that you use can affect your skin dramatically, so you need guidance before you make a purchase. Take protective measures for sensitive skin and buy products that treat the symptoms of psoriasis while minimizing outbreaks.

## ◈ Bye-Bye Age Spots! How to Treat Hyperpigmentation

Hyperpigmentation is another skin disorder that has many different looks, ranging from common age spots and freckles to larger areas of hyperpigmentation known as melasma. Hyperpigmentation can be an embarrassing problem, spurring people to search for more effective treatments to minimize the appearance of the darker patches.

There are many options in treating hyperpigmentation, from complex cosmetic procedures at the doctor's office to simple home treatments applied topically to the skin. We will take a look at some of the home treatments that allow sufferers to enjoy a brighter, more even complexion.

## Exfoliation

One of the most effective ways to treat hyperpigmentation is with exfoliating treatments. While your doctor has a plethora of options such as microdermabrasion and chemical peels, these procedures usually cause some discomfort and have a significant recovery time. The good news is that you can perform exfoliating treatments right at home. While home products do not penetrate as deeply as professional exfoliation treatments, they are sufficient in minimizing the appearance of hyperpigmentation, particularly if they are used regularly.

One company that offers effective home peel products is Actifirm. Actifirm Z-Peel comes in two different concentrations for home use, allowing people of every skin type to take advantage of its exfoliating benefits. Actifirm Z-Peel uses unique ingredients like the extracts from Japanese mushrooms and a variety of other botanicals to create a thorough exfoliation product. Treatments are completed in just a few minutes, and repeated sessions will provide stellar results.

## Effective Ingredients

Another way to treat hyperpigmentation is through the use of key active ingredients with a demonstrated ability to lighten skin. When looking for a skin lightener, it is important to read the labels before purchasing a product. Look for skin lighteners with ingredients like hydroquinone and Kojic acid, which have proven through testing to have a positive impact on hyperpigmentation when used regularly. If your skin care product doesn't list proven, active ingredients, it probably won't give you the desired results.

Kojic acid and hydroquinone are additives in Neostrata's Intense Lightening Complex. This formula comes in gel form, and it has shown excellent results in treating hyperpigmentation when used regularly. There are also hydroxy acids in the product that offer mild exfoliating benefits and cell turnover during the lightening process. The formula balances skin tone for a beautiful complexion.

For those whose skin is sensitive to ingredients like hydroquinone, there are other options available. One natural substance that also has a positive impact on hyperpigmentation is green tea extract. This ingredient is found in Cellex-C's Fade Away Gel for Sun and Age Spots. In addition to green tea extract, this formula includes the patented Cellex-C complex that provides a host of skin benefits. The product contains an SPF 25 to protect the skin from sun damage while treating the current hyperpigmentation.

Hyperpigmentation can be an embarrassing problem, but there are many options for treating this skin condition. If age and sun spots are interfering with your lifestyle, consider a topical solution and enjoy lighter, brighter skin without a trip to the doctor's office.

## Photo-rejuvenation for Treating Hyperpigmentation

Photo-rejuvenation uses laser light (also called Intense Pulsed Light or IPL) to remove the first few layers of skin in order to eliminate hyperpigmented areas and reveal the clearer, lighter skin underneath. Photo-rejuvenation using IPL can also lessen the appearance of rosacea (a reddening of the skin), balance skin tone, repair minor sun damage, increase skin elasticity, and improve overall appearance. IPL has also been effective at reducing pore size. IPL is non-invasive and is recommended for patients with extremely sensitive skin who cannot withstand microdermabrasion or more intense laser therapies.

Photo-rejuvenation treatments take 45 to 60 minutes each and may require several sessions. They are relatively painless procedures, but for patients with extremely sensitive skin, the physician may apply a topical anesthetic cream to reduce pain. This is applied 15 to 30 minutes before the actual treatment begins. After treatment, there may be a temporary increase in reddening, and hyperpigmented areas may even appear slightly darker, but over the course of a few days, these conditions will diminish and dark spots will lighten significantly.

Photo-rejuvenation usually requires five to seven treatments performed every four to six weeks. Pregnant women, epileptics, or people taking cortisone or steroid injections should avoid Photo-rejuvenation.

If you decided to pursue Photo-rejuvenation to treat your hyperpigmentation, make an appointment with a physician who can safely provide this therapy. The first step is a pre-consultation to determine whether you are a good candidate for Photo-rejuvenation. The best candidates are those with light skin. You'll also discuss the number of treatments that will be necessary to achieve the desired results and have a patch test. Be prepared to pay for the patch test that is performed to make sure that you can tolerate photo-rejuvenation. If the patch test is negative, you can arrange your first appointment.

Hyperpigmentation is a very treatable skin condition, and Photo-rejuvenation is a safe and effective way to address it.

## ❖ UNDERSTANDING AND CONTROLLING ROSACEA

If you have a blush that never seems to go away, chances are you have a skin condition called rosacea. Rosacea is quite common for fair-skinned people between the ages of 30 and 50. Many things can trigger rosacea, so it is essential to know some of the causes in order to control the condition.

In the United States alone, approximately 14 million people have rosacea. It most often affects adults between the ages of 30 and 60. It is more common in women. A condition called vascular rosacea causes persistent flushing and redness. Blood vessels under the skin of the face may dilate, and show through the skin as small red lines. There is no exact cause of rosacea, but several different opinions exist.

## What Triggers Rosacea?

While there are many things that can cause blood to rush to your face, that does not necessarily mean you have rosacea. If, however, the redness is from small, very visible blood vessels then you may have rosacea.

## ❖ Emotions

Stress and anxiety play a major role in causing rosacea. When you are angry or upset, chances are your face reflects your emotions and becomes red and flushed. Sudden changes in emotion can trigger episodes such as crying, laughing, yelling or euphoria. If you are called on in public or are suddenly embarrassed by some situation, you may demonstrate your anxiety by flushing.

## ❖ Food and Drink

Spicy foods or foods that are very hot when consumed may cause the face to flush. This holds true with hot drinks like tea or coffee as well. Alcohol definitely causes rosacea to flare, especially if you're a heavy drinker. The simple answer, of course, is to avoid the foods and beverages that trigger flare ups, or at least minimize their consumption in order to keep rosacea under control.

## ❖ Activities

Activities that cause extreme exertion such as running, lifting or any type of exercise that increases your breathing levels can cause rosacea. Regardless of whether you are working or playing, if you have rosacea, strenuous activities can make your skin flush. One way to minimize the problem is to schedule two shorter work-out periods instead of a single, long session. Hold work-out sessions when and where it is cooler, and drink lots of water to stay hydrated. Limit hot baths, hot showers, and trips to the saunas to decrease the chances of an occurrence of rosacea — bathe in temperate water instead.

## ❖ Weather

Weather plays a big part in aggravating rosacea. It doesn't matter if it is hot weather or cold since both can trigger an occurrence. Humidity can also be a trigger if you perspire a lot. If you're exposed to the sun or wind, you may experience flushing. Using sunscreen when you are outdoors or anticipate any exposure to the sun is essential if you need to control rosacea and prevent sun damage.

## ❖ Medical Conditions and Medications

Women going through menopause may experience rosacea, but this could be temporary due to the hormonal changes they're experiencing. A chronic cough or a cold can trigger rosacea as can withdrawal from caffeine or other addictive substances.

Medications such as blood pressure medicine, topical steroids, and pain killers may all act as triggers. Talk to your physician about medications to avoid if you suffer from rosacea.

## ❖ Other Triggers

Certain skin care products may antagonize existing rosacea and could even cause an initial outbreak. It is important to understand the products you use, and whether they are appropriate for people with rosacea. Seek advice from a dermatologist or skin care professional to ensure that you are using the correct products for your condition.

## Some Relief

There are treatments available for rosacea that include antibiotics and skin care products designed to help the problem.

**B. Kamins Rosacea Starter Kit** – The B. Kamins Rosacea Starter Kit is a great option for traveling since it contains all of your favorite products in smaller, travel friendly sizes. The B. Kamins Rosacea Starter Kit Includes:

❖ Booster Blue Rosacea Cleanser 2 fl. oz

❖ Booster Blue Rosacea Treatment 0.5 fl. oz

❖ Booster Blue Rosacea Masque 1 oz

❖ Sunbar Sunscreen fragrance-free 1 fl. oz

**NeoStrata Sensitive Rosacea Prone Protocol** — This product is formulated with PolyHydroxy Acids (PHAs, gluconolactone, and lactobionic acid) which are non-irritating, natural humectants that bind with water and increase moisture production in the skin. PHAs also strengthen the vulnerable protective barrier in the skin, making it less sensitive to irritants. As a potent anti-oxidant, PHAs help prevent environmental and oxidative damage. Lactobionic Acid also helps support collagen so skin has a more youthful fullness and elasticity. In clinical studies, PHA regimens reduced redness and provided powerful anti-aging benefits without irritation, even in patients with atopic dermatitis and rosacea.

# ❦ 7 ❧

# NATURAL ANTI-AGING SKINCARE

F or many years, people have been waiting for the latest, greatest scientific breakthroughs in skin related products, for new synthetic chemicals and processes that would help them miraculously turn back the clock. Yet natural products have proven to be the most effective and healthiest products that you can put on your skin. The movement toward natural products follows the trend in health care in general, as more and more health care practitioners realize the strengths and advantages of using all-natural ingredients in products that affect all of the body's systems and organs. Natural ingredients have the strength to achieve the results that we desire, with far fewer side effects than synthetic, chemical compounds.

A wealth of natural ingredients are now included in skincare products. The use of vitamin products has been extremely effective in both helping to reduce the appearance of age-related skin conditions and in slowing the aging process. The vitamins in many skincare products are extracted from sources we consume in our everyday diets, such as fruit and vegetables. Vitamin C and E have both proven to be powerful ingredients in natural skincare products.

Natural ingredients are also drawing more and more heavily on antioxidants. Antioxidants are chemicals that destroy free radicals, harmful chemical compounds that range through the body, destroying cells as they go. However, there are several thousand different types of antioxidants and free radicals, and some antioxidants are more effective at destroying certain types of free radicals than others. By finding antioxidants that target the free radicals specifically responsible for causing aging effects, scientists can create natural skincare products to target and destroy those free radicals. This methodology has led to the creation of some exceptionally powerful, and effective, natural skincare products.

By finding antioxidants that target the free radicals specifically responsible for causing aging effects, scientists can create exceptionally powerful, and effective, natural skincare products.

Natural skincare products are much less likely to cause irritation to sensitive skin. People with sensitive skin may find that their skin becomes irritated when products with harsh chemicals or those with artificial perfumes and dyes are applied.

## ❖ NATURE MEETS SCIENCE: MARINE EXTRACTS IN SKINCARE

Beauty from the sea is not a new concept; Cleopatra herself was known to bathe in the mineral-rich Dead Sea to preserve her youthful allure. However, as science has learned more about how and why the sea benefits our skin, companies have begun to explore the use of marine extracts in their own products. The result is a plethora of choices in marine-based skincare, designed to soften the skin, prevent the signs of aging, and treat a host of skin disorders.

## Rich in Minerals

Marine extracts are often rich in minerals like copper, zinc, and iron. These substances are useful to the skin because they help hold in hydration so the skin does not become dry. The moisturizing effects of these ingredients often last much longer than other types of hydrating substances, leaving the skin feeling soft and smooth between treatments. Algae extracts are particularly useful for this purpose. A high mineral content stimulates blood flow throughout the body, leaving skin that is not only smoother but healthier as well.

## Anti-Aging Properties

The anti-inflammatory properties and antioxidant content of marine extracts makes them a good choice in anti-aging skincare products. The substances found within marine extracts may stimulate the production of collagen and elastin, which may result in firmer, plumper, and younger-looking skin.

## Treatment Options

For those with a number of skin conditions including acne, psoriasis, and eczema, marine extracts can by the key to smoother skin. Some marine extracts control the amount of sebum produced by the body. While our skin needs a certain amount of sebum to remain soft and healthy, too much can result in skin conditions like acne. By controlling sebum production, you can be sure that your skin is getting all the nutrients it needs to remain soft, smooth, and breakout-free.

One skincare line that makes good use of both marine extracts and scientific breakthroughs is Ageless Derma Stem Cell and Peptide Anti-wrinkle Cream. Its formulas include pure marine extracts to generate the greatest benefits.

# Natural Remedies for Slowing the Aging Process

It is important to keep the skin well hydrated and moisturized to ward off the visible signs of aging like wrinkles, fine lines, and dry skin. Hydration starts from the inside out so drinking lots of water throughout the day can keep the skin well hydrated and help it maintain the proper balance necessary to deter the aging process. Skin cells that are well moisturized are plumper, firmer and suppler. Many natural skincare products contain moisturizing ingredients like natural oils, honey, aloe vera, herbs, and citruses. Many also help diminish fine lines and wrinkles while still others aid in controlling acne and other skin conditions.

## ❖ ESSENTIAL OILS AND OTHER INGREDIENTS

Many natural skincare products include ingredients that have been used to care for the skin for thousands of years. Most of these oils penetrate easily and deeply into the skin to revitalize it and keep it moisturized and replenished. The most common essential oils found in natural skincare products are oils from olives, soybeans, coconuts, almonds, sesame, castor beans, and grape-seed. Many people still use these oils at home by applying them to warm, moist skin right after a shower or bath.

Many ingredients are found in natural skincare products, but the ones that are most beneficial to the skin include hyaluronic acid, which helps restore, repair, and lock collagen and elastin together and keep them bound to prevent further breakdown. Green Tea Extract and citrus fruits like lemon, lime, and orange all work well to reduce fine lines and wrinkles. If you look at the ingredients in the products you purchase, you will find that most of them contain these extracts and use them in various quantities so that your skin can be restored to its natural, youthful look with a radiant glow.

## ◈ NATURAL BEAUTY USING PHYTOTHERAPY AND AROMATHERAPY

With concerns over the many synthetic substances and chemicals we apply to our skin and put into our bodies today, people are turning away from manmade products and looking for effective, natural solutions for better health. This is particularly true in skincare, and top quality companies are expanding their research to determine the most effective natural solutions for treating a host of skin conditions and concerns.

Scientists are finding that many botanicals and other natural ingredients provide even better treatment options than the synthetic formulas used in the past. Let's take a look at the role phytotherapy and aromatherapy play in skincare today.

### What is Phytotherapy?

Phytotherapy is a methodology that uses plants, as well as their extracts and essences, to treat a host of ailments. Phytotherapy has been used for medicinal purposes for centuries.

Today, phytotherapy is a popular philosophy in many skincare products, providing a natural solution to skin issues like acne, sun damage, and the effects of aging. The key to effective phytotherapy is the use of plants in their purest forms, allowing for the use of the highest possible concentrations without the damage usually caused by the extraction process.

## What is Aromatherapy?

Aromatherapy is another methodology that has been practiced for centuries. It involves using essential plant oils to enhance one's physical and mental well being. Essential oils can be inhaled or applied directly to the skin in diluted concentrations to produce a host of desirable effects.

Aromatherapy is frequently used in skincare products, both to provide a pleasant scent when the product is applied, and to enhance the effectiveness of the formula. The method used for extracting the oil from the plant is important, as is the combination of essential oils with other natural ingredients that provide the greatest benefit.

The products that we apply influence the beauty of our skin. When you combine phytotherapy and aromatherapy in natural, effective formulas, the results are usually softer, more radiant skin.

### ◈ THE BEST NAMES IN NATURAL SKINCARE

One effective way to keep skin looking its best is by indulging in natural skincare. Natural skincare never includes chemicals or synthetic ingredients in the mix. Instead, formulas are crafted with botanicals and other natural ingredients for skin that is clean, soft, and young looking. For some, this means mixing combinations at home, but many companies today make excellent commercial products that use only natural ingredients. We will take a look at some of the top names today.

**Yonka** — Yonka has been synonymous with high quality, natural skincare since the company began in 1954. Yonka was founded by three French brothers with a passion for using botany in skincare formulas. This trio introduced aromatherapy and phytotherapy to the natural skincare market along with a collection of Mediterranean essential oils that became the basis for their collections. The company is still family owned and operated, with clients all over the world enjoying the benefits offered by the natural skin-care line.

**Bioelements** — Unlike Yonka, Bioelements is a relative newcomer to the natural skincare scene. This company was started in 1991, by an esthetician who was interested in creating top quality skincare products for both professional and home use. The advantage of Bioelements products is that they provide the same effective ingredients in your home skincare regimen as you would receive in the salon. Formulas are carefully blended with the most potent ingredients available to address everything from the early signs of aging to the occasional acne breakout.

Bioelements uses both botanicals and scientifically engineered ingredients to create effective formulas. There are no artificial dyes or fragrances in any of the Bioelements natural skin-care products.

**Pevonia Botanica** — Pevonia Botanica is another natural skincare company that takes its responsibilities a step further. In addition to restricting its formulas to high quality botanicals and organic extracts, this company conducts none of its research on animals and ensures that all of its manufacturing practices are environmentally friendly. This commitment filters right down to the biodegradable packaging used for all of its products. This company never uses harmful substances like parabens or artificial dyes in any of its products. The lines are specially blended to suit each specific skin type for best results. Products are available for every age, skin type, and gender.

**Nuxe Paris** — Nuxe Paris is a skincare company that uses a combination of phytotherapy and aromatherapy in their skincare lines. This European company uses high quality ingredients and pure extraction methods to create a highly effective formula. An average of 80% of Nuxe ingredients are of natural origin. This company has been creating skincare products since 1957. Nuxe offers a wide range of skincare options, including products specifically designed to turn back the clock. The company also provides body products that leave your skin feeling soft and smooth.

Natural skincare used to take hours in the kitchen, whipping up formulas with ingredients found right in the pantry. While you can still find effective natural skincare recipes, many people prefer the convenience of commercial products with equivalent combinations. Thanks to companies like Yonka, Bioelements, and Pevonia Botanicals, you can find high quality, all natural skincare in formulas that are ready to use. Natural skincare products are the perfect choice for treating your skin firmly but gently in order to obtain the most beautiful results.

# ❧ 8 ☙

# The Science Behind the Ingredients

## ◈ Familiarize Yourself with Key Ingredients

With the wide number of anti-wrinkle products being advertized every day, many of us have become familiar with the names of key ingredients, but we have no idea what they actually do. You may wonder exactly what Retinol, lanolin, polyphenols, and Coenzyme Q10 are. Which ones are right for your skin's needs? Before buying, do some research on the effectiveness of the various ingredients used in anti-aging products and the percentages of active ingredients included. The percentages should be the most important factor you consider when choosing anti-aging skincare products. Due to the high cost of active ingredients, most anti-aging skincare products don't contain enough of them to be effective.

Consider the following questions prior to making a purchase:

❖ Do the ingredients stimulate skin regeneration or renewal?

❖ Are they present in an amount that will actually be effective?

❖ Do any of the non-active ingredients interfere with the effectiveness of the active ingredients?

❖ Are any ingredients potentially harmful to the skin?

A little research and forethought will make you less susceptible to the latest industry gimmicks and help you make an informed decision about the anti-aging skincare that is best suited to your needs.

## ◈ WRINKLE CREAM WITH HYALURONIC ACID

Hyaluronic acid is a carbohydrate found naturally throughout the body. It works to keep the joints and muscles lubricated. Unfortunately hyaluronic acid has a short life span—about one day on the skin. This means it must constantly be replenished to keep the skin nourished. If the skin has enough hyaluronic acid, its collagen will continue producing the connective tissue that keeps the skin structured and toned, leaving the skin firmer and more youthful looking.

Like many other things in the body, hyaluronic acid production diminishes as we age. It leaves collagen with less moisture, and this collagen starts to sag and dry out because it cannot maintain the level of hydration needed to stay supple. This leads to wrinkles and other aging problems that will continue to worsen if the hyaluronic acid levels in the skin are not increased.

## Why the Skin Needs Hyaluronic Acid

The skin is where 50% of the body's hyaluronic acid is stored. It is found in all layers of the skin and keeps the skin moistened by binding as much as 1000 times its weight in water. Collagen in the skin keeps it firm and hydrated so that when the skin stretches. it returns to its original shape.

Besides retaining water and providing nourishment to the skin, hyaluronic acid is also used to reduce inflammation and is vital to keep the skin looking and feeling healthy. Skin without this vital ingredient begins to look tired, loose, wrinkled, and unattractive. It can also cause premature aging if not treated. Hyaluronic acid has been successfully used in products to treat conditions like psoriasis, melasma, and rosacea, and it has also been effective when used for acne, anti-aging, and discoloration of the skin or scarring.

## Where to Find Hyaluronic Acid

Since our production of hyaluronic acid reduces with age, we need to find ways to replenish our supply so that we can repair the skin that has been damaged through environmental stress and sun damage or premature aging. Hyaluronic acid is found in many skincare products because it is a great moisturizer and extremely beneficial to the skin. There are many anti-aging products available that contain hyaluronic acid including creams, cleansers, lotions and many other products, but the amounts of hyaluronic acid in these products vary tremendously, so you need to read labels carefully to determine which one is right for you.

Health supplements are another way to replenish hyaluronic acid. These are taken internally rather than applied topically to the skin. Some supplements with ample amounts of hyaluronic acid may be more expensive than others, especially those that are injected rather than taken in capsule form. You can find these hyaluronic acid supplements in pharmacies, vitamin shops, or health food stores; they can also be found online through distributors or online stores.

## Are There Side Effects of Hyaluronic Acid?

Most topical products in the forms of creams, lotions, cleansers, masks, or other treatments won't contain high concentrations of hyaluronic acid but, as noted, the concentrations will vary by product. Few people have a negative reaction to hyaluronic acid, but it could cause a mild reaction like a rash or minor skin irritation that will disappear when you stop using the product. If the hyaluronic acid is injected into the skin, it could cause redness or slight pain for a while but there are rarely any long-term allergic reactions. You should not take hyaluronic acid (especially by injection) during pregnancy or if you are breast feeding as the effects to the infant are unknown at this time.

## ◈ ALPHA HYDROXY ACID CAN MAKE YOUR SKIN GLOW

Alpha Hydroxy Acid is an ingredient found in many skincare products, but what you probably don't know is that it has been used to keep the skin looking young since the time of the ancient Egyptians. Alpha Hydroxy Acids or AHAs, as this group of compounds is known, include glycolic, malic, citric, tartaric and lactic acids. You will find Alpha Hydroxy Acid in many foods such as sugar cane, wine grapes, citrus fruits, apples, and sour milk.

Today Alpha Hydroxy Acid is found in products such as facial creams, sunscreen, shampoo, skin lightening products, and products formulated to control acne. They are used in many different concentrations for chemical peels, microdermabrasion, and other facial treatments that are performed in a physician's or a dermatologist's office.

These treatments have much higher Alpha Hydroxy Acid concentrations and are deemed more effective; however, the procedures are also more expensive than self-administered, over-the-counter products (OTC). The OTC products consumers use at home generally contain about 5% concentrations, and never more than 10%.

# Benefits of Alpha Hydroxy Acid

The ancient Egyptians knew that alpha hydroxyl acid could reduce wrinkles and fine lines and other visible signs of aging. It can also exfoliate and remove dead and dry skin cells that tend to make the skin appear dull and lifeless, increase the blood flow, and renew the skin's cells so they are energized. AHA is also used for lightening skin or evening out skin tones. It is often used to address hyperpigmentation or brown spots caused by aging or sun damage. It will reduce blackheads and can help control acne outbreaks.

Skincare products for at home peels contain AHA and are an inexpensive way to refresh your skin yourself with a minimum of effort; however, the low concentrations in the OTC products may provide only limited results, making additional applications necessary. True results may take as long as 6 months to be realized.

If you have a chemical peel or other treatment in a physician's office, the down time is longer. Skin takes time to heal and it may look like you have experienced a bad sunburn for a few days, but the end results can be amazing. With the higher concentrations used in the doctor's office, you will see immediate results with a reduction or disappearance of wrinkles and fine lines, and the effect can last up to five years, making it a good value for the money.

## Skin Types are a Factor

Your skin type has a great deal to do with how high a concentration of Alpha Hydroxy Acid your skin can handle. The OTC products are considered safe for people to use at home, but people with sensitive skin or those prone to rosacea, dermatitis, or other skin disorders might experience unwelcome itching, stinging, or a slight rash. If this occurs, stop using the product and seek a physician's advice.

If you do use AHA products at home, remember that they are designed to be used on a daily or weekly basis depending on the product. You must be patient, because it may take months to see any real improvement in wrinkles and fine lines. Everyone's skin is different, so the results will vary by individual. While using these products, it is important to remember to use a sunscreen during the day as you do not want to subject the new skin to any sun damage.

## ◈ BEAUTIFUL SKIN RELIES ON THE POTENT ANTIOXIDANTS IN GREEN TEA EXTRACT

For centuries, the Chinese used green tea extract in medicines and as remedies for ailments like headaches or indigestion. Green tea extract has become extremely popular due to its known therapeutic values. It is used extensively in skincare products because its potent antioxidants combat the free radicals that cause skin damage and are a primary cause of aging.

Whether you drink green tea or purchase products that contain it, there seems to be ample proof that it promotes good skin health and makes you look younger. This is good news for anyone serious about keeping their skin healthy and looking young.

### Benefits of Green Tea Extract

With its rich supply of antioxidants, green tea extract has antibacterial properties that make it very effective at stimulating the immune system. It is an effective treatment for acne, helps heal the skin, and keeps it protected during the healing process. It reduces inflammation and works synergistically with sunscreen to neutralize the sun's rays. When using green tea extract, be sure to use a zinc oxide-based sunscreen to avoid unwanted chemical reactions.

Green tea extract rejuvenates skin cells and repairs them so that their life cycle is extended with regular use. It has been used to treat skin conditions like psoriasis, rosacea, and acne through the regeneration and soothing of irritated, inflamed, and wounded skin. It has been very effective in controlling acne without any of the adverse side effects that are often found in similar products. It has even been suggested that green tea extract prevents skin cancer by blocking the harmful enzymes that cause it.

## Look for Products with Genuine Green Tea Extract

Though green tea extract is a powerful antioxidant, it becomes less potent when it comes in contact with oxygen. It is important to ensure that the green tea extract product you purchase contains the concentrations needed so it can work its magic on your skin. If it is genuine, then green tea extract should be one of the first ingredients listed on the label. It might also be listed as EGCG or catechins. Concentrations should be 200 milligrams or more to be effective. Anything less will have little effect.

If green tea extract is positioned near the bottom of the ingredient list, chances are there is very little green tea extract in the product. If the label reads "green tea fragrance", it is not what you are looking for— green tea needs an essential oil to be able to penetrate the skin. Look for the carrier oil to see what has been used to dissolve the green tea extract. These could include herbal extracts, oils, or alcohols. Camellia oil is derived from green tea and is considered one of the best carrier oils, but it is also expensive, so it is rarely used.

## ❖ FLAWLESS SKIN USING COENZYME Q10

Most skincare products contain Coenzyme Q10, but what is this odd sounding ingredient? Coenzyme 10 is a vitamin that produces energy in the skin. You can actually get Coenzyme Q10 from some of the foods you eat like salmon, soybeans, or spinach. It is a vitamin made naturally in the body but production declines as you age. Savvy skincare companies put it in their products to replenish what your body no longer produces.

## What Does Coenzyme Q10 Do?

Coenzyme Q10 is an antioxidant that combats free radicals. Coenzyme Q10 limits the damage free radicals can do, which makes it a key ingredient in anti-aging products. It ensures that the skin retains vital moisture and prevents damage to the collagen and elastin that could otherwise cause the skin to become thinner. Coenzyme Q10 keeps skin plump and cells healthy and moist.

## When to Start Using Coenzyme Q10

Our bodies start losing optimum levels of Coenzyme Q10 by the time we reach 30, so it is important to start taking measures to replenish this important antioxidant early in life.

You won't see an immediate difference when you start using skincare products with Coenzyme Q10, but you will start to notice an improvement within about six weeks. The important thing is that you are taking defensive measures against free radicals and taking proactive steps to reduce wrinkles and other signs of aging by using skincare products with Coenzyme Q10 listed as an ingredient.

You will find Coenzyme Q10 in face and eye creams and other anti-aging treatments or serums. You'll also find it in body products and even cleansers. Be sure to look for the quantity of Coenzyme Q10 and ensure you are getting at least 200 milligrams per day—particularly those of you in your 50s. Take active steps early and you'll soon be on the road to flawless, radiant and youthful looking skin.

## ◈ HYDROQUINONE IS THE RIGHT SOLUTION FOR HYPERPIGMENTATION

Hydroquinone is a chemical complex—crystalline in form—that is often used in skincare products to remove pigmentation. It is also known as quinol and has a scented base that is used in over the counter products with concentrations of 2% or less. Concentrations higher than 2% require a prescription from a physician.

## Melanin and Skin Pigmentation

Pigment in the skin is called melanin. Melanin protects the skin against UV rays, but excessive exposure to the sun or scarring may cause an overproduction of melanin, the darkening the skin. People with lighter skin have less melanin than people with darker skin, which is why Caucasians require more sun protection than someone with dark skin.

## Treatment for Hyperpigmentation

People with skin conditions like hyperpigmentation, age spots, or sun damaged skin may want to take steps to even out their skin tones. Hydroquinone is one of the most popular ingredients used to bleach or reduce discoloration in the skin. It is a dynamic bleaching agent that retards or stops melanin production while breaking down any existing melanin.

## Types of Products

Hydroquinone is often found in bleaching or skin lightening creams or lotions that are designed to be used over time. It is an easy way to bleach the skin, and it can be done at home without the need for dermabrasion or other treatments that are more time consuming and costly. These hydroquinone creams are a convenient and cost effective way to treat spots that can worsen if left untreated.

## Use of Hydroquinone

Before using Hydroquinone, you should test a small amount on your skin to see if it causes any reaction or irritation to the skin. Cleanse the area thoroughly, apply the cream to the designated area, and massage it gently into the skin. For best results, apply it to a dark area you plan to treat as it will lighten normal skin. Always wash your hands thoroughly after each application. Hydroquinone cream is applied twice daily and you usually see results in approximately three weeks, although actual results could take up to four months. Timelines vary with each individual.

## Are There any Side Effects?

Some people experience skin irritation that usually clears up on its own when they discontinue using the product. Side effects could include redness, itchy skin, other types of dermatitis, or allergic reactions. If the condition continues or you develop other symptoms like crusty skin or swelling, contact a physician immediately. Do not use hydroquinone if you are pregnant or breast feeding. Hydroquinone should not cause a reaction when used with other medications you may be taking, but consult your physician if you have any questions about compatibility.

## ◈ Kojic Acid is a Natural Treatment for Hyperpigmentation

Many people suffer from hyperpigmentation caused by skin disorders such as acne, eczema, or allergic contact dermatitis. It can also be caused by excessive exposure to the sun, normal aging, birthmarks, or freckles. Whatever the cause, hyperpigmentation can be very unattractive especially on the face as it causes uneven skin tones that are sometimes difficult to cover with makeup. In Japan, kojic acid has been used extensively as a skin lightener for hyperpigmentation.

### What are the Benefits of Kojic Acid?

Kojic acid is currently used in many skincare products that bleach or lighten the skin. It is a topical treatment found in creams, lotions, and soaps. The concentration level is usually 1% to 4%; higher levels can cause irritation to the skin. While a good product for reducing freckles and age spots, kojic acid might not be the best choice for more pervasive levels of hyperpigmentation

### Where Do You Get Kojic Acid?

Kojic acid is naturally derived from a fungus and blocks the enzyme tyrosinase—an important element in the production of melanin. Kojic acid combats and stops the production of melanin right at its root and counteracts the antioxidant properties of tyrosinase, thereby reversing excessive darkening of the skin.

You can buy kojic acid in its raw form, but that is not recommended, as it may cause damage to the skin if not diluted in a gel or cream. Although the Japanese safely consume kojic acid in their daily diet, it can cause irritation when used directly on the skin. Skincare products containing kojic acid can be found in department stores, skincare stores, and online.

## Side Effects of Kojic Acid

Overall, kojic acid is very effective as a whitening agent to bleach the skin or reduce brown spots and other hyperpigmentation issues, and it is found in many skincare products formulated for this purpose. It is also used in some food products. It has been known to cause mild to severe skin irritation in some people and excessive use can cause contact dermatitis for people with some skin types. This may manifest as itchy skin, a rash, or redness. Kojic acid can become unstable if exposed to air or sunlight so some products use a compound kojic dipalmitate that is more stable but less effective.

Often kojic acid is combined with other ingredients to aid in the lightening process and to minimize skin irritations. For example, vitamin C is often combined with kojic acid to provide more even skin tones and protection from the UVA and UVB rays of the sun.

## Recommended Usage of Kojic Acid

Before using skincare products with kojic acid, you should consult a dermatologist to discuss your hyperpigmentation issues and create a treatment strategy. You should always use a broad spectrum sunscreen when you use any kojic acid products as they may make the skin more sensitive to the sun and hyperpigmentation could worsen without protection.

Kojic acid cream should only be applied to areas of hyperpigmentation, or darkened areas of the skin. It can have an undesirable effect if used on normal skin. Allow the kojic acid cream to absorb into the skin completely before applying any other product or makeup on top of it. Kojic acid skincare products take time to produce visible results and may take up to six months or more to deliver the lightening effects you are looking for. If any skin irritation occurs, you should stop using the product immediately and contact your physician or dermatologist for advice.

## ❖ SKINCARE PRODUCTS WITH RETINOL REDUCE WRINKLES

Retinol is one of the most common ingredients in good anti-aging creams. Studies have shown that Retinol can diminish fine lines and wrinkles, and it also helps promote the production of collagen to keep the skin firm and plump.

## What is Retinol?

Retinol is a chemical in the retinold group and a form of vitamin A. The retinold compound also includes tretinoin, a prescription only anti-aging ingredient. Retinol is popular because it can be bought over the counter without a prescription. It is also able to permeate the skin to connect with the elastin and collagen that lie beneath the surface. Vitamin A is essential to collagen and elastin to keep the skin taut and firm.

## Skin Damage from the Environment

Skin that has been exposed to the sun and other environmental stressors like smog, pollution, or smoke becomes damaged over time. Damaged skin begins to lose collagen and elastin, and so loses its elasticity and firmness, allowing wrinkles and fine lines to creep in and make us look older. Skincare products with retinol can help counteract these premature aging factors.

## Retinol has Many Good Uses

Mature and aging skin is often very dry, because moisture in the skin is not being replenished as it should be. Retinol is a good moisturizer as it rehydrates the skin and ensures that the skin oils are at their proper levels. Anti-aging creams with retinol reactivate the skin cells that have become dormant, giving skin a wake-up call and enhancing cell growth leaving your skin with a more rejuvenated look.

Regular use of a retinol cream tightens the skin so that the texture is smoother, softer, more youthful, and refreshed. This is because as skin cells continue to multiply and regenerate, wrinkles and expression lines start to disappear. Retinol is an excellent exfoliator and has been very effective in the treatment of acne and blemishes.

## What to Watch Out For

Regular use of a retinol cream could cause some mild irritation or itching if your skin is very sensitive, but this is a normal reaction and is usually temporary. Retinol skincare products should be used in the evening, because they make the skin more sensitive to sunlight. If you use retinol cream during the day, you should always use a sunscreen to protect your skin. If you experience any type of lasting irritation or problems with your retinol cream you should stop treatment for awhile and see a physician if the irritation persists. Sometimes, an anti-aging cream with a lower percentage of retinol may be recommended for people with more sensitive skin.

## ◈ PSP ANTI-AGING SKINCARE: USING PROCESSED SKIN CELL PROTEIN TO TURN BACK TIME

The field of anti-aging skincare is constantly evolving with new products and ingredients being introduced onto the market all the time. One skincare company has developed an entirely new approach to anti-aging skincare using cultured fetal skin cells to produce processed skin cell protein. Processed skin cell protein, also known as PSP, helps the skin obtain an optimum balance of nutrients for younger looking skin.

### Neocutis: Paving the Revolution

Neocutis is the company responsible for this new technology. It is a Switzerland-based skincare company with offices in San Francisco, and it obtains skin cells from a Swiss cell bank that provides skin tissue to heal wounds and treat conditions like psoriasis and eczema. However, the technology is now turning to the anti-aging industry, with a line of restorative skin creams and serums designed to turn back the clock.

The theory behind the treatment is that the skin takes a beating over the years, due to:

❖ Damaging sun rays

❖ Air pollutants

❖ Home pollutants

❖ Harmful chemicals

❖ The natural aging process

❖ Modern cosmetic procedures

Bio-restoration is often necessary to restore youthful vitality to the skin. It rebalances the skin's nutrients, heals damaged skin, and rejuvenates dull complexions.

At this time, Neocutis is the only company offering anti-aging products containing PSP. There has been some controversy over how fetal skin cells are obtained at the beginning of the process, leading many companies to shy away from the technology. However, skin cells have been used for some time to treat skin conditions and injuries. Neocutis is simply taking the process a step further by using PSP for cosmetic reasons.

## Uses for Processed Skin Cell Protein

While the technology is still relatively new, there are many potential benefits associated with using PSP in anti-aging products. These include:

❖ A reduction in the appearance of fine lines and wrinkles

❖ Improved firmness in the skin

❖ Enhanced skin texture and tone for a younger, more radiant look

Neocutis has performed clinical trials to prove the effectiveness of its formulas. The results of the trials are posted on the company website. Studies have shown that aging skin has needs similar to those of wounded skin. It stands to reason that skin cells that generate growth and balance to heal injured skin will also work effectively to reverse the effects of aging. At this time, Neocutis products are only available in the United States through health care professionals.

Talk to your physician if you are interested in trying products that take full advantage of PSP. Neocutis offers a wide line of skincare products containing this ingredient. The products also include a host of other moisturizing ingredients designed to plump and hydrate the skin from the outside in.

## ◈ RADIANT SKIN COMES FROM VITAMIN C – A POTENT ANTIOXIDANT

We have been told that vitamin C is good for us, but did you know that it is also a potent antioxidant that helps to protect and provide many benefits to the skin? Most people want to have skin like they had when they were young—soft and smooth and radiant! You can have that radiant skin with the help of vitamin C, which you can find in many different skincare products and in capsule form.

Vitamin C is so prevalent in skincare products because it offers so many good things for your skin. Let's take a look at some of the ways that vitamin C helps your skin stay fresh and radiant.

**Collagen production**—Collagen is needed to keep the skin taut and firm, but as we age, the skin produces less of this vital protein, causing wrinkles and fine lines to appear. Vitamin C is essential to the production of collagen.

**Moisturizer**—Vitamin C actively helps the skin to keep hydrated.

**Exfoliation and cleanser**—Vitamin C helps with exfoliation—the removal of dead skin cells—and clears pores of excess oils and debris. This in turn keeps the skin healthy and looking radiant.

**Softener** — Vitamin C helps soften the skin, making it smoother and more refined.

**Antioxidant** — Vitamin C is an antioxidant that protects the skin and prevents the growth of melanin which results in dark spots caused by exposure to the sun. However, vitamin C does not block harmful UV rays, and so sunscreen should always be worn during the day to avoid more damage to the skin.

## Vitamin C by Other Names

If you look carefully at skincare product labels, you will almost always see vitamin C listed, but it may appear in different forms. Here are some other forms of vitamin C that you may find in skincare products.

**Magnesium ascorbyl phosphate** — This is a derivative of vitamin C that is becoming more and more popular because it is more stable and less acidic than vitamin C itself. Note: unless your skincare product has a high concentration of Magnesium Ascorbyl Phosphate, it will not enhance the production of collagen.

**Ascorbic acid or L-ascorbic acid** — This is often used in exfoliates to remove dead skin cells and debris. It is the basic form of vitamin A from citric, acid but it should not be used directly on the skin, particularly if the skin is sensitive, because it will irritate.

**Ascorbyl palmitate** — This is the most common derivative of vitamin C. It is used in skincare products because it is not as acidic as pure vitamin C.

**Tetrasubstituted lipophilic ascorbates** — These are becoming more popular as they are less expensive than other forms of vitamin C and seem to be just as effective in the production of collagen — a big plus.

Vitamin C continues to be a viable and important skincare ingredient that boosts the production of collagen and exfoliates the skin. New derivatives of vitamin C are constantly being introduced to the market, and they are delivering promising results, but those results vary by product and user. Regardless, the future looks bright for these vitamin C derivatives as many of them have the attributes of vitamin C but are more stable and cause less irritation to the user.

## ◈ SOLID RESEARCH SUGGESTS COPPER PEPTIDES FOR ANTI-WRINKLE SOLUTIONS

Copper peptides activate the natural processes of repair and renewal in the skin, hair, and nails. Clinical studies have shown that copper peptides are effective in restoring and rebuilding the skin's collagen production and removing collagen and elastin that has been damaged beyond repair.

### What are Copper Peptides?

Copper peptides are small fragments of proteins that attach themselves to copper, creating a compound that aids in the regeneration of tissue. Proteins are building blocks that are essential for living tissue like skin. They are especially effective in healing wounds and other types of skin lesions. They reduce the formation of scar tissue and stimulate normal skin restoration. They are also effective in anti-aging products as they enhance the production of collagen and elastin and, in turn, firm the skin, reduce unwanted wrinkles, and remove fine lines.

### What are the Benefits of Copper Peptides?

Because of their ability to trigger regeneration, copper peptides are becoming more popular in skin and hair care solutions. They are also increasingly used after treatments such as chemical peels, dermabrasion, and laser resurfacing to improve and encourage recovery and healing.

Copper peptides are proving effective at enhancing the production of collagen, making the skin firmer, smoother and tauter. Copper peptides also enhance the thickness of the epidermis and dermis of the skin and encourage skin cell regeneration in otherwise thinning skin.

Copper peptides can also reduce blemishes and blotchy skin while improving the skin's elasticity by thickening the fat layer. Copper peptides have an anti-inflammatory property that is effective in healing wounds or other skin lesions and in reducing scar tissue. They stimulate skin restoration so that it returns to its normal look, and also reduce irritation associated with treatments and wounds to maximize healing.

## Are There any Side Effects with Copper Peptides?

Copper peptides skincare products are considered very safe. They have been subjected to a series of thorough tests to scrutinize their effectiveness. The amount of copper is usually only about 0.1%. This means that if you follow the manufacturer's instructions, you should have few if any side effects. While some people may experience mild skin irritations such as a rash, redness, or itching, any side effects are usually temporary and clear up if you stop using the product. Symptoms of excessive copper in the body might include dizziness, headache, weakness, and fatigue. Be extremely careful when using copper peptides products around the eyes. Overuse in this delicate area could lead to loose or sagging skin—the opposite of what you are trying to achieve.

## Getting Effective Results with Copper Peptides

Using products containing copper peptides will not provide immediate results. It is a slow process that could take many months since the skin only renews itself every 30 days or so. This means that you should plan a regimen that is easy to follow. Exfoliate the skin on a regular basis so that dead skin cells are removed and new skin emerges. Use an on-and-off schedule with copper peptides to give your skin a chance to regenerate naturally and rest between treatments.

### ❖ THE BENEFITS OF ALPHA LIPOIC ACID

Alpha lipoic acid (ALA) is a fatty acid produced naturally by the body and found in some of the foods that we eat. It is both fat and water soluble, so it can be found in your muscles and internal organs in varying degrees of concentration. ALA plays an important role in our metabolism, converting carbohydrates into energy.

The production of ALA in the body helps create energy, but in large concentrations, it can also become a powerful antioxidant that combats the many free radicals that cause harm to the body and the skin. ALA also helps regenerate other antioxidants such as vitamin E and vitamin C.

## ALA Production Diminishes with Age

As we age, the amount of ALA produced by the body decreases. Taking ALA supplements helps keep free radicals under control. These supplements are often used to treat diseases and conditions such as diabetes, cataracts, glaucoma, cancer, strokes, vascular diseases, and HIV. ALA is not a drug, so it is not regulated by the Food and

Drug Administration, but it is often found in skincare products because it is a potent antioxidant.

## How ALA Affects the Skin

Although there are no clinical studies that support ALA as a treatment for anti-aging, it is often touted as effective in decreasing the visible signs of aging like fine lines and wrinkles. It seems to improve the texture of the skin by inhibiting the cross-linking of proteins that cause wrinkles and harden the arteries.

The beauty of ALA is that it is much more powerful than many vitamins, including vitamins E and C, because it can penetrate both oil and water and so works both outside and inside the body to make other vitamins more efficient, provide protection, and rebuild skin cells that have been damaged by environmental stressors.

Alpha Lipoic Acid is one of the body's most important antioxidants that fights environmental stress and protects it from further onslaught. ALA is beneficial because it reduces stress while helping other antioxidants to combat skin conditions, visible signs of aging, and other harmful or degenerative diseases. It is a hard worker that, when used in conjunction with other vitamins and antioxidants, keeps the body and skin protected at all times.

## ◈ INGREDIENTS TO LOOK FOR IN ANTI-WRINKLE CREAMS

When it comes to anti-aging creams and other skincare products, everyone is looking for a quick fix that will reduce wrinkles or fine lines otherwise known as crow's feet or expression lines. We are aging every day, and many of us do not know how to rejuvenate our skin, yet there are hundreds of products out there all advertising that they help you do just that. So where do you begin? Let's look at some of the ingredients found in these products so you can narrow your search and determine what you need.

**Allantoin** — Aids in the repair and regeneration of skin cells. It has healing and anti-inflammatory properties and helps smooth the skin.

**Alpha-hydroxy acids (AHA)** — Contains glycolic acid that exfoliates, repairs and enhances the skin. It stimulates the production of collagen, increases the thickness of the skin, improves elasticity and texture, and smoothes skin tone. It can also minimize enlarged pores and provides an effective way to treat acne.

**Argireline** — An ingredient used in some anti-wrinkle cosmetic products that are on the market. These products are applied directly to the skin. Argireline is the trademark name for the molecule acetyl hexapeptide-3. Argireline is made up of a chain of six amino acids or proteins. It is similar to Botox, but the Argireline peptide string is shorter than that of Botox.

**Beta hydroxy acid or salicylic acid** — Used to enhance the tone and texture of oily skin. It is often used to treat acne as an alternative to AHA. Concentrations should be 1-2% to be effective.

**Coenzyme Q-10** or **Co-Q10** — An antioxidant that repairs skin damaged by the sun. It stimulates new skin cell growth. It increases the firmness of the skin and smoothes the texture.

**DMAE** — Effective in minimizing wrinkles and fine lines and firming sagging skin. It enhances hydration and is often used along with other vitamins.

**Green tea** — Used as an antioxidant to help heal the skin, while it reduces puffiness and minimizes inflammation. Often used in moisturizers, it reduces large pores, wrinkles and fine lines.

**Hyaluronic acid** — Clinically proven to reduce wrinkles and fine lines. Use it with vitamin C to increase absorption into the skin.

**Hydroquinone** — Used as a skin lightener to reduce dark spots and hyperpigmentation. It effectively bleaches the skin to create an even tone. Concentrations should be 1-2% to be effective.

**Kinetine** — This ingredient is marketed under the brand name Kinerase. It is often used on sensitive skin to decrease fine lines and wrinkles and enhance skin tones. Generally used around the eyes, concentrations should be 0.1%.

**Kojic acid** — A clinically proven treatment for lightening hyperpigmentation or brown spots. It deters the production of melanin in the skin. It is an alternative to hydroquinone.

**Liposomes** — Effective in reducing wrinkles and fine lines while enhancing the texture of the skin. They are also used to provide nutrients directly to skin cells.

**Matrixyl 3000** — Developed by the Sederma Corporation, this ingredient is made up of the matrikines peptides Pal-GHK (palmitoyl oligopeptide) and Pal-GQPR (palmitoyl tetrapeptide-7). They work together as antioxidants to fight the damaging signs of aging on the skin. Together they stimulate the matrix molecules (collagens and fibronectin), which in turn allows the Matrixyl 3000 to reduce wrinkles. It is distributed as a gel with a pH of 4.0-6.0, and 30% water content.

**Palmitoyl pentapeptide or Matrixyl** — Enhances the production of collagen and helps repair skin damaged by the sun. It also reduces wrinkles and improves elasticity so the skin is firmer. It is an alternative to retinol.

**Retinoic acid or retin A or tretinoin** — Although it can cause irritation, it is the strongest form of vitamin A used to treat skincare issues. It reduces wrinkles, increases the production of collagen, exfoliates, and smoothes the skin while improving elasticity and reducing the occurrence of acne.

**Retinol** — Another form of vitamin A, it is not as effective as Tretinoin because it does not absorb well into the skin. It may cause skin irritation.

**Retinyl palmitate** — A vitamin A derivative similar to Tretinoin, but it is milder so it won't irritate the skin.

**Syn®-Coll** — This is an effective and needle-free alternative to collagen injections. This product is a small peptide that mimics the body's mechanisms to produce collagen. *In vitro* testing showed that Syn®-Coll increased collagen synthesis by 119%. It was then tested on a control group of 60 healthy volunteers who applied it as a cream twice daily. They the saw wrinkles improve more than 350% after 84 days of use as compared with the group using a placebo cream.

**Vialox** — A potent anti-wrinkle ingredient that has proven to reduce wrinkling by 49% by limiting the contraction of muscle cells. It is similar to Botox, but is a topical cream rather than an injection, making it attractive to people who are squeamish about injections on the face.

**Vitamin C or ascorbic acid** — Increases production of collagen, heals the skin, and has potent antioxidant properties.

**Vitamin E or tocopherol** — An antioxidant that protects and heals the skin. It is effective in treating dark circles under the eyes. It can also be used to treat bruises and broken capillaries.

## ◈ Which Ingredients Do the Best Skin Lightening Products Contain?

People seek skin lighteners for a variety of reasons, including age spots, freckles and sun damage, but what, exactly, is in these products? Many of the ingredients found in skin lighteners are natural derivatives, but it is important to know just what you are getting when you purchase a product to help lighten your skin.

**Alpha-arbutin** — Another natural ingredient derived from the leaves of bearberry plants, it can also come from cranberry, blueberry and pear leaves. It works in conjunction with beta-arbutin to block melanin production.

**Avocado oil** — Used in cosmetics for its moisturizing effects, it is also known to reduce age spots, lessen sun damage, and reduce scarring.

**Beta-arbutin** — A white powder that comes from the leaves of a bearberry plant originating in China. It is primarily used to minimize liver spots and freckles or to treat sunburn.

**Extrapone nutgrass** — Derived from a root found in India, it inhibits melanin and is very effective as a natural skin lightener or whitener. It also reduces freckles.

**Gigawhite 5%** — This is a skin brightener. With regular use, it brightens the skin, reduces age spots, and corrects melasma within two to three months. It is a plant extract useful for both oily and dry skin types.

**Glycolic acid 10%** — Derived from the sugar cane plant, it exfoliates the skin, balancing uneven tones.

**Hydroquinone** — This is a powerful skin whitener. In the United States, concentrations are limited to 2% in over-the-counter products, and 4% in prescription products.

**Kojic acid** — Stops melanin (dark pigment) production and minimizes the appearance of liver spots, freckles, acne, and pregnancy spots. First found in mushrooms in Japan, it is used in very small amounts in skin lightening products to offset possible negative side effects.

**Mulberry extract 0.5%** — This natural derivative functions as an antioxidant, helping improve the skin's metabolism and purity. It can help whiten skin, lessen the appearance of freckles, increase skin flexibility, and deter wrinkling.

**Niacinamide 5%**—This is a combination of vitamin B3 and niacin. It has anti-inflammatory effects, making it useful for skin conditions such as acne, dark spots, uneven skin texture, and red blotches.

**Retinol**—This is a form of vitamin A. It resurfaces and smoothes the skin and gives a more youthful look. It penetrates the skin on a deep level and helps produce a glowing complexion.

**Tyrostat**—This plant extract inhibits the tyrosinase enzyme that creates red or brown pigmentation. Tyrostat is a skin whitener that is very safe and effective.

## ◈ THE INGREDIENTS TO LOOK FOR IN EFFECTIVE CLEANSERS

With so many skin cleansing products available on the market these days, it's important to know a little about what these products contain. Some skin cleansers work better than others, depending upon the stated ingredients, so it makes good sense to educate yourself a bit before you buy. Read the labels on cleansers to see what the ingredients are. What does each ingredient do for you? Here is a list of the most widely used ingredients found in today's natural cleanser market.

**Almond oil**—This is an emollient that lubricates the skin, making the product easy to massage into the area. It nourishes and provides a proper moisture balance on the skin's surface.

**Aloe vera**—Widely used for medicinal reasons, aloe vera is an effective product for burns, sunburn, and skin infections. It adds a unique aromatic moisturizing effect to skin cleansers.

**Alpha hydroxy acid (AHA)** — This is a chemical compound found in nature or created in a laboratory. It increases collagen production and thickens the skin without causing inflammation. It exfoliates and is found in over-the-counter concentrations of 5%-10%. Higher concentrations may be used by physicians to treat extreme acne, dark spots, and fine wrinkles. Multiple treatments may be necessary for long-lasting effects.

**Retinol** — This is a form of vitamin A found in animals. Its main benefit is that it diminishes fine wrinkles and tightens skin for a more youthful appearance. It can also exfoliate and slough off dead skin cells.

**Resveratrol** — This plant derivative is a strong anti-inflammatory agent. It helps clear the skin and boosts the natural turnover of skin cells. Resveratrol moisturizes and refreshes the skin, giving a more youthful appearance. It is particularly good for skin prone to blemishes.

**Shea butter** — This is a completely natural ingredient found in soaps. It is extracted from the nut of the shea tree, found in Africa. It can be eaten and is sometimes used as a substitute for cocoa butter. It melts at 98.6°F and is absorbed into the skin without leaving a greasy feel. The most effective level in cleansers is 5%-7%.

**Tangerine oil** — This is just what it implies: the oil expressed from the tangerine fruit. It increases blood circulation to the skin, giving it a clear, radiant look. It also helps treat acne. An added benefit is that it also has a wonderful citrus aromatherapy effect.

**Tea tree oil** — Taken from the leaves of a plant found in Australia, tea tree oil can fight against staph infections and MRSA. At 5%, the ingredient can be used to treat acne, dandruff, and dry skin. It is very effective as a skin treatment when coupled with aloe vera.

# ◈ THE INGREDIENTS YOUR EXFOLIATOR SHOULD CONTAIN

We all want fresher, younger-looking skin, and you can achieve that glow of youth no matter what your age. Exfoliating the skin sloughs off dead skin cells and gives your skin a fresh start. There are several ways to exfoliate. You can rub the skin with a towel or brush, with a facial cream, a peel, a mask, or a body scrub, but using chemical products and creams means you need to sort through a huge variety of products to find the one that is right for you. Here are the key ingredients you should look for when purchasing a skin exfoliator.

**Alpha hydroxyl acid (AHA)** — These glycolic and lactic acids can take years off the skin's appearance. They are often found in chemical peels. Over-the-counter products must contain less than 8% AHA, but professionals may use concentrations up to 30%. If you don't find the actual percentage listed on the label, it should appear as the second or third ingredient in the list. AHA eases fine lines, removes surface scars, and gives a more youthful look to the skin. It should be noted that, when used in the higher concentrations, AHA can cause redness and flaking that may last for weeks. It is best used on normal to dry skin.

**Glycolic acid** — A form of alpha hydroxy acid, glycolic acid can penetrate the outer skin layers and is often used by dermatologists in chemical peel treatments. Concentrations for over-the-counter use should range from 10% to 20%.

**Papaya extract** — It is rich in vitamin C, potassium, and vitamin A. This fruit extract exfoliates dead skin cells, aids in the repair of damaged skin, and clears up other skin problems. It also helps speed up chemical reactions. Only a small amount is needed.

**Retinoic acid** — This is a vitamin A product that can help reduce lines and wrinkles. It stops pores from becoming clogged with dead cells, improving skin texture and brightness. This ingredient helps with skin renewal by increasing skin thickness and stimulating new collagen formation. Care must be taken when used on delicate or sensitive skin.

**Retinyl palmitate** — This is a form of vitamin A. It stimulates new skin cell production, plumps the skin, and increases collagen. It has sunscreen and anti-oxidant properties.

**Salicylic acid** — This is a compound found in plants that is often used to treat acne. It works to open clogged pores and encourages new skin cell growth. It also helps prevent bacteria from entering the skin cells. It is best used on normal to oily skin and skin prone to blemishes. This ingredient is often used in dandruff shampoos to help exfoliate the dead skin cells on the scalp and prevent further dryness.

**Shea butter** — This is a natural fat extracted from the nut of the shea tree. It is used to moisturize and has healing properties. It keeps skin soft and helps maintain flexibility.

## ◈ SEARCH FOR THESE INGREDIENTS IN YOUR SKIN TONER

Toner should be an important part of your daily skin cleansing routine. We all want to look fresh and have our skin feel smooth and taut. When you purchase a skin toner, you want to know that you are buying the best product you possibly can. A good toner will cleanse your skin, reduce the size of pores and help tighten the skin, giving you a more youthful, fresher appearance. You'll want a product that can decrease any puffiness and even out your skin tone, especially when used on your face. The ingredients you should be looking for in a toner are listed below.

**Aloe vera** — This is derived from a succulent, cactus-like plant. It is an anti-inflammatory, stimulates cell growth, and repairs damaged tissues. It also gives skin a healthy glow and moisturizes it.

**Chamomile** — This is a flower, much like the daisy. It helps with the healing and regeneration of skin cells. It also has anti-inflammatory properties and is an anti-oxidant. It helps reduce puffiness and cleanses the pores.

**Centella asiatica** — This is great at improving circulation in the skin. It also helps build collagen and makes the skin firmer and more elastic. It can also minimize varicose veins and broken capillaries.

**Cranberry** — This fruit has huge anti-oxidant effects on the skin. Cranberry helps fight infections that can originate from air pollution, cigarette smoke, and other outdoor and indoor elements. It is also rich in vitamin A which helps with pigmentation, and skin color, and tone.

**Grapefruit seed extract** — This has deep cleansing properties. It helps fight bacteria, parasites, fungi, and viruses. It works as an astringent and boosts circulation. It should be diluted to at least 2%.

**Horse chestnut** — The active ingredient in this extract is escin, which helps improve circulation and has anti-inflammatory properties. Horse Chestnut helps prevent vein and capillary leakage that can cause swelling of the skin. It contributes to having healthier collagen overall.

**Jojoba** — This is actually a liquid wax but it is very similar to the oil found in human skin, and is used to moisturize. Extracted from the seed of the jojoba tree, it helps balance the skin's production of oil.

**Vitamin B5** — Also called pantothenic acid, this ingredient helps decrease pore size. This vitamin repairs damaged tissues and smoothes the skin. It also combats acne by aiding in the regulation of skin oils.

**Yarrow** — This is an herb (also known as Ladies' Mantle) that helps fight inflammation. It helps even out the skin tone through the use of its astringent properties. It can also be useful to fight infection and helps the body get rid of toxins that can aggravate the skin.

## ❖ INGREDIENTS NOT TO USE IN SKINCARE

When checking the ingredients on skincare products, note that there are certain substances that should not be used at all, and some that don't add any value to the product's efficacy. Some of these ingredients can actually cause problems like pimples. Here are some ingredients to **avoid**:

**Alcohols** — Alcohol, when listed as an ingredient in skincare products, should be avoided. Alcohol is a drying agent. It causes the body to lose water, not keep it. It can cause red areas on the face, similar to rosacea, as it dilates blood vessels. These dilated blood vessels can become permanently damaged with continued use of alcohol-based products, giving the skin an unattractive reddish, flushed color.

**Dioxane-1, 4** — Dioxane may be found in trace amounts in certain cosmetics and skincare products. It is not used as an actual ingredient, but can be formed as a byproduct of other ingredients during the manufacturing process. Manufacturers are not required by law to disclose the use of 1, 4-Dioxane on their ingredients label. Skin absorption studies performed by the Food and Drug Administration have found that Dioxane is absorbed through the skin when it is contained in skin lotions. Dioxane is an issue in baby shampoo and lotions as it is a possible carcinogen.

**Fragrances** — Many skincare products contain fragrances which can be inhaled or absorbed through the skin. The ingredients that make up fragrances are not usually listed on the cosmetic container due to a loophole in the law allowing "trade secrets" as they apply to fragrances. There may be quite a few secret or hidden ingredients contained within the product, many of which contribute to the aroma. Some of the ingredients in these scents can be toxic, especially to women who are pregnant. Certain chemicals can disrupt hormonal balance, sending up red flags for cancer concerns. Some people are allergic or very sensitive to many fragrances, so using them in skincare products puts not only the user at risk, but also those with whom they come in contact as they are subjected to secondhand scent. Allergic reactions can include contact dermatitis, headaches, and asthma symptoms. Fragrances that contain hormone disrupters have been linked to thyroid problems, sperm issues, and even cancer.

**Mineral oil** — Mineral oil is an emollient, a petroleum byproduct — it is not oil made from minerals as the name implies. Skin moisturizers containing mineral oil trap water under the skin by forming a layer of oil on top of it. Used in excess, it can turn the skin too white, soggy, or soft. Mineral oil used in skincare products, especially when used in industrial strength strains, causes pimples and blemishes on the face. The oil can clog pores, leaving the skin unable to release toxins through the sweat glands. It is also possible that mineral oil may be a cancer-causing agent.

**Parabens** — These are preservatives found in many cosmetics, moisturizers, and hair care products. The most commonly used parabens are methylparaben and propylparaben. They have been linked to breast tumors due to their estrogen-like properties.

## ಬಂ 9 ೞ

# LOOK AND FEEL YEARS YOUNGER WITH FDA-APPROVED, NON-SURGICAL COSMETIC PROCEDURES

R ecent breakthroughs in non-invasive, anti-aging laser technology have made it possible to erase years from your age without costly surgical procedures and with a minimum of downtime. According to the International Spa Association, non-invasive cosmetic procedures have tripled in the last five years. We will discuss some of these non-invasive procedures in this chapter.

## ◈ DERMAL FILLER

Dermal fillers are usually performed in a doctor's office or a Medical Spa. The filler is injected into the area that needs to be plumped or filled in. People may opt for dermal fillers for a variety of reasons. They fill in facial lines and wrinkles, correct nasolabial folds, reduce the appearance of acne scars, and correct other dermatological problems. The substances used for each of these problems may vary but, in each case, the goal is to make the skin look smoother by filling the area out with collagen or other soft tissue materials. While dermal fillers can be very expensive, the effect can last for up to three years.

Some of the most well known dermal fillers are Botox and Restylane. Other injected substances include Radiesse,

Juvederm, Perlane, Zyplast, Zyderm, Dermalogen, Artecoll, Hylaform and Dermalive. Each of these will be discussed in detail to provide a useful guide for you when you get ready to choose a dermal filler.

## ◈ BOTOX

Botox has been used clinically for various purposes since 1989. It is actually a purified version of botulinum toxin, a bacterial substance used to treat various problems including muscle disorders. It decreases muscle activity by blocking the release of acetylcholine. Given in tiny doses and injected directly into the muscles that lie underneath a wrinkle or line, it weakens and relaxes the muscle, giving the skin a smooth surface at the injection site. The results can last for up to three months. People usually choose Botox to decrease facial lines such as crow's feet, frown lines and other facial impressions. It has been one of the most common non-surgical cosmetic procedures since 2005 when more than eight million procedures were performed in the United States alone.

## Advantages of Botox

A Botox injection only takes about thirty minutes to administer and causes very little, if any, discomfort. The final effect is a smoothing of the wrinkled area and a more youthful look. Botox is most effective at alleviating lines and wrinkles on the upper third of the face. It corrects the lines between eyebrows, frown lines, and wrinkles around the eyes. It can be used together with other wrinkle fillers for an even more effective outcome. When injected into the lower eyelid, it gives a wide-eyed look that many women desire. Injected into the bottom of the nasal septum, it can give one that "ski-slope" appearance to the tip of the nose.

# Disadvantages of Botox

Because Botox does not last for more than three to five months at a time, regular maintenance is necessary to keep up the desired appearance. This can be expensive, with treatments running upwards of five hundred dollars each. It may take as much as four weeks for the desired results to take full effect, quite a long wait for some people. There are also possible side effects from the use of Botox. Some patients have experienced droopy eyelids, a result of the muscle being so relaxed that it cannot lift itself. Other common side effects are headaches and some nausea. Less often, patients may experience weak muscles, pain at the injection site, inflamed and tender areas of the skin or muscle, and swelling at the injection site.

## ❖ ARTECOLL

Artecoll is a soft tissue injectable filler that is very long-lasting or permanent. It is used to correct wrinkles and reduce nasolabial folds which can become prominent with age. Artecoll can also treat deep wrinkles between the eyebrows, lines in the corners of the lips, and lines on the upper lip.

Artecoll is mainly composed of collagen. A quarter of the product is made up of microscopic plexiglass beads (polymethylmethacrylate or PMMA), and the rest is bovine collagen. The PMMA is what gives Artecoll its long-lasting results. PMMA has been used in the medical field since 1945. It has been used to make dental prostheses and hip implants, in cranial surgery, and for many other procedures. It has been used as tissue filler for over twenty years. Zyplast injections, which are a simple form of bovine collagen without PMMA, are used in a similar manner to Artecoll, with Artecoll producing slightly better results.

Artecoll is injected beneath the dermal layer, into subcutaneous fat. A second treatment may be needed after three months. It must be injected properly, at the correct angle, in order to prevent lumps from forming under the skin. The ideal age for treatment is between forty and fifty years old, when clients have lines they want corrected but believe it is too early to consider a drastic solution, such as a facelift.

## Advantages of Artecoll

Studies have shown that the majority of patients treated with Artecoll are satisfied with the results and would recommend the injections to other people. In fact, most report that they would repeat the procedure. Most patients feel little or no pain as the substance has a small amount of the anesthetic lidocaine built into the solution.

## Disadvantages of Artecoll

A skin test to determine possible allergic reactions is usually suggested with Artecoll. Schedule the test about two weeks before treatments begin, as bovine collagen can cause adverse reactions. This, of course, delays the beginning of treatment for patients. Possible negative side effects reported after receiving Artecoll injectable fillers include an undesirable firmness in the area treated, increased sensitivity at the site, and persistent pain. Patients who receive Artecoll injections may also develop granulomas, large lumps under the skin. They may develop up to fourteen months after receiving Artecoll treatment and can be difficult to treat or correct. Even when treated, the nodules may continue to reappear indefinitely.

## ◈ DERMALIVE

Dermalive is a permanent dermal filler composed of non-animal ingredients: hyaluronic acid, hydrogel hydroxyethylmetacrylate (HEMA), and ethylmetacrylate (EMA) co-polymer particles. It was first used in France and other European countries in 1998. Dermalive's primary use is as a cosmetic filler for lines and wrinkles. It is similar to Artecoll in that it also contains polymer particles. Both HEMA and EMA ingredients have been clinically proven to be safe and are widely used for making various types of medical implants. The high water content in HEMA becomes trapped inside the acrylic molecules (EMA), making the injected substance very elastic and flexible.

Dermalive is used to correct very pronounced nasolabial folds, smooth facial lines and wrinkles, and to fill in acne scarring and other indentations affecting facial contouring without the need for surgery. Patients can add volume to cheeks, cheekbones, and skin using Dermalive. It is injected inside the dermal layer, just below the line or wrinkle to be corrected. The skin's volume plumps to meet the outer layer and smoothes the skin's surface.

The substance, once implanted, is permanent, non-biodegradable, and is usually well tolerated, although some adverse reactions are still possible. In the months following the procedure, the body generates new collagen fibers naturally. This production of collagen then surrounds the acrylic particles, filling the area more completely and creating younger-looking skin and a smoother facial area.

## Advantages of Dermalive

Dermalive gives a patient long term results, from five to ten years for most, much longer than temporary injectable fillers. Because of this, touch-up sessions are few and far between. Patients are usually able to achieve a very natural, smooth appearance with the use of Dermalive. This filler has a low incidence of negative reactions.

## Disadvantages of Dermalive

Granulomas or lumps under the skin may form as much as two years after being treated with Dermalive. These must sometimes be surgically removed. Patients may need one or two additional injections in order to achieve the best effects permanently or semi-permanently. Mild pain may be felt at the injection site, but this can be mitigated with the use of a topical anesthetic. There may be redness or swelling at the site. The treatments are expensive, with the price of one treatment averaging between $900 and $1,000

### ❖ HYLAFORM

Approved by the U.S. Department of Agriculture in 2004, Hylaform is an injectable dermal filler used to treat moderate to severe wrinkles. Some of the most common facial lines and wrinkles treated with Hylaform are deep furrow frown lines on the forehead and between the eyebrows, smile lines on the corners of the mouth, and nasolabial folds from the bottom of the nose leading to the mouth. It can be used to augment thin lips often associated with aging, to correct deep acne scarring, and to fill other facial contours. The formula fills the space between the skin's collagen and elastin fibers. This brings the skin back to the more youthful look it had before wrinkles or scarring set in.

Hylaform is made up of hyaluronic acid, a substance contained in human skin and that of other mammals; Hylaform is taken from the combs of roosters that are bred for this purpose. It is offered in gel form and is clear, odorless, and injectable.

## Advantages of Hylaform

In general, no skin test is necessary for Hylaform treatments, as it is a substance already found in the body. Hylaform injections are easy, painless, and give immediate results. The effects of Hylaform are long-lasting, up to one year for some people. This dermal filler is a bit more affordable than Restylane or Botox, and it can give similar or better results. The procedure for injecting Hylaform takes less than thirty minutes on average. Because Hylaform is a naturally-occurring body substance, no dangerous residue is left in the body. This injectable filler is naturally absorbed by the body.

## Disadvantages of Hylaform

Side effects usually associated with Hylaform injections are mild episodes of redness, swelling, or bruising. Although prior allergy testing for the substance is not required, patients allergic to birds need to be informed of the composition of the filler. Patients may encounter a slight stinging sensation at the injection site. Also, granulomas, or lumps, may occur under the skin and may require surgery to remove. If patients are using Hylaform for lip augmentation, they may experience increased sensitivity in that area. Swelling and redness may occur, but it should normalize within hours.

## ◈ JUVEDERM

Juvederm is an injectable dermal filler gel used to soften facial wrinkles and deep folds in the skin. It is mostly hyaluronic acid, much like Restylane, Dermalive,

Hylaform, and other fillers. Hyaluronic acid is a naturally-derived substance found in the skin, tendons, and muscles of humans and other mammals. It promotes fullness and volume beneath the skin's surface. Injections of Juvederm fill the spaces between collagen and elastin fibers in the skin, renewing volume and making the patient look younger. Removing and smoothing nasolabial folds or "smile lines" is the primary use for Juvederm. In fact, in studies comparing Juvederm with Zyplast (another popular dermal filler), 80% of the patients using both products found Juvederm to be more effective at smoothing facial folds. This filler gel is also often used as a lip augmenter and as filler for facial scarring.

## Advantages of Juvederm

Juvederm is one of the longer lasting dermal fillers with a single treatment often lasting up to a year. Juvederm injections cause less bruising and inflammation than with some of the other dermal injectables. Juvederm is also more comfortable, because it contains the anesthetic lidocaine. Juvederm offers little risk of hyperpigmentation or hypertrophic scarring, making it safe and effective for persons of color. Because Juvederm is a hyaluronic acid and a naturally occurring human substance, there is little chance of an allergic reaction. Minor reactions like redness seldom last more than a week.

As with all dermal fillers, the effect of Juvederm is temporary; this is good in that it gives patients a chance to see if they actually are happy with the results. Juvederm is reabsorbed into the body through normal digestive processes. If the proper look is achieved, patients may opt to receive future injections; if they are not happy with the results, they can do nothing and allow the skin to return to its former condition.

## Disadvantages of Juvederm

Although this substance works well, it is reabsorbed into the body within six to nine months, making repeat injections necessary to maintain the desired effects. This can get costly. Users may notice some bruising, redness, soreness, swelling, and bumps at the injection site. Juvederm is not recommended for people with severe allergies.

## ◈ PERLANE

Perlane, a cosmetic dermal filler, is useful for smoothing moderate to severe facial wrinkles and lines around the eyes, nose, and forehead. It is also used to augment or plump lips, repair facial depressions, and help fill in acne scars. Perlane's active ingredient, hyaluronic acid, is a natural component found in human connective tissues.

Hyaluronic acid is the body's natural way of adding fullness and volume to the skin. It is an injectable gel and can be molded to fit different contours.

Perlane injections take about thirty to forty-five minutes to administer and should only be given by board certified physicians such as a dermatologists or plastic surgeons with experience using dermal fillers.

## Advantages of Perlane

Because Perlane is a naturally occurring substance, there is no skin test necessary prior to use. There is little or no threat of allergic reaction to this dermal filler. Results can be expected to last up to a year, which is longer than many cosmetic fillers on the market. Perlane can also be used in combination with Botox for even better results. There is very little pain associated with Perlane injections;

however, some patients may want a pre-applied topical anesthetic to ease the pinch of the injection.

## Disadvantages of Perlane

Because Perlane is a hyaluronic acid, it is broken down by the body and depleted over time. It is a temporary solution for lines and wrinkles. This treatment is costly; sessions cost $500 to $900. It is usually more expensive than Restylane, another similar treatment. Perlane's most common side effects are swelling, redness, and bruising at the site of injection Also, small bumps of the gel may become visible beneath the skin; however, these should reduce with time. The gel tends to increase the build-up of natural collagen in the body. It is not recommend for people with severe allergies to bacterial proteins.

## ◈ RESTYLANE

Restylane is used to plump the folds and lines on the skin's surface. It is made from a non-animal hyaluronic acid. Water binds with this acid, producing a more voluminous look to the skin's surface. A dermatologist or other qualified practitioner injects the product quickly and with ease. Often there is no anesthetic required. When Restylane is injected into the dermis, it fills the spaces between the aged fibers of collagen and elastin; this helps renew the volume lost with age.

Restylane is most often used as a lip plumper. It is injected just below the skin's surface, into the tissue of the face. Very much like Botox, Restylane is also useful for filling lines and wrinkles, such as crow's feet, eye creases, and lines on other wrinkle-prone areas of the face. It is also useful for adding volume to the cheeks and shaping the chin, forehead, and nose.

## Advantages of Restylane

There is no risk of infection with the use of Restylane. Restylane is a natural substance; therefore there is little fear of an allergic reaction. It is not an animal by-product or a completely synthetic substance like some of the other dermal fillers. Depending on the size of the area to be treated, injections may be spaced over the course of ten minutes to an hour. When an anesthetic is used, it is a local anesthetic or numbing agent only. The needles used to inject the product are very thin, causing little discomfort. You will see an immediate plumping effect, ridding the face of lines and wrinkles. This effect can last for up to twelve months; they fade gradually but last much longer than other dermal filers. Patients can return to normal activities immediately after receiving injections. Restylane gives excellent, positive results that last for months.

## Disadvantages of Restylane

Although allergic reactions are rare, those with any specific bacterial allergies or known reactions to hyaluronic acid should avoid the product. There may be a temporary reaction at the injection site such as swelling, inflammation, discoloration, or tenderness.

You need repeated injections of the substance in order to maintain the desired look, but patients can go for much longer periods between injections than they can with other dermal fillers. This is not a permanent solution to wrinkles and lines.

### ◈ ZYDERM

Zyderm, similar to Zyplast, is a plumper, adding volume and smoothing lines and wrinkles. Collagen is the main ingredient of Zyderm. The dermis, just below the skin's outer layer, is made up of collagen, which is critical to cell and blood vessel growth.

Zyderm actually behaves as a reinforcing structure for the skin, helping hold everything in place. It replaces some of the depleted natural collagen with collagen produced from cows (bovine). Zyderm is injected into the dermal area just under the skin using a very fine needle. The human body adapts easily to this protein injection. Zyderm is manufactured in two forms: Zyderm I, used to correct fine lines, wrinkles, and superficial scarring. Zyderm II is for more severe lines and scarring on thicker skin.

## Advantages of Zyderm

Results are seen quickly and the injections are relatively painless because Zyderm contains the anesthetic lidocaine. This is particularly beneficial for lip augmentation, because there are so many nerve endings in the lips. Treatments start at about $300 for small areas, which is comparatively inexpensive compared to other fillers. Any swelling or bruising usually subsides within days.

## Disadvantages of Zyderm

The effects of Zyderm only last about two to three months, and then repeat injections are needed to maintain results. Because Zyderm comes from cows, it may cause an allergic reaction in some people. Patients should take a trial skin test (usually done on the patient's arm) at least four weeks before any actual treatments are started. The skin test may cost up to $150. Possible reactions include swelling, redness, pain, and small bumps under the skin.

## ◈ ZYPLAST

Zyplast is a collagen dermal filler. Zyplast helps counteract the signs of aging by replenishing the skin's collagen and drawing fluid (water) to the treatment area. It works by lifting or adding volume to the skin's depressions. It is often used for plumping lips. Purified bovine collagen, which has been in use in the United States for the past thirty years, is the main active ingredient in Zyplast. The filler is cross-linked with an organic compound known as glutaldehyde. This combination makes Zyplast last longer and allows it to be used on more severe scars and wrinkles. The collagen in Zyplast is injected right along the edges of the lines, scars or wrinkles using a very thin needle.

## Advantages of Zyplast

Zyplast is long-lasting, making wrinkles less noticeable for up to a year. The injections are not painful as the substance has an anesthetic built into it. A topical anesthetic can also be used before application if desired. The injections take about fifteen minutes for each area treated.

## Disadvantages of Zyplast

Because Zyplast is not naturally occurring like hyaluronic acid, skin testing must be done about four weeks prior to actual treatments in order to predict any possible allergic reactions. This extends the time patients must wait to achieve actual positive results. Reactions to Zyplast include burning or stinging in the area being treated. There may also be some bruising, swelling, and/or tenderness in the injected area, and small bumps may form under skin, but they are temporary. Zyplast injections cost

$300 to $500 depending upon the size of the area to be treated and the amount of filler needed. Although Zyplast can last many months, it does wear down over time.

## ◈ Dermalogen

Dermalogen is filler derived from the skin tissue of human donors. It has been processed using techniques similar to those used for organ transplants. Any infectious agents are removed from the product during processing. It is similar to collagen in its ability to correct lines and wrinkles.

Dermalogen is primarily used to treat facial contour defects such as those found in nasolabial folds. It is very effective for correcting depressed scars caused by trauma, surgery, or acne by elevating the depressed areas to the same level as the skin surrounding it. It compares favorably with other injectable dermal fillers. It can be used for filling nasolabial folds, lines around the eyes known as crow's feet, lines on the forehead such as horizontal or vertical frown lines, wrinkles, and for nose and eyelid reconstruction. It can be combined with Botox to maximize effects, particularly in the upper facial areas. Dermalogen is also often used in conjunction with laser skin resurfacing, chemical peels, or facial surgery.

## Advantages of Dermalogen

The use of Dermalogen as an augmentation filler is popular and safe. There is no allergy testing required before using Dermalogen, and there should be little inflammation after use. The positive effects can last longer than those derived from bovine collagen fillers. The positive effects of Dermalogen increase with each treatment, giving patients more noticeable improvements after every session. This filler looks and feels natural and is pliable and soft to the touch.

## Disadvantages of Dermalogen

The injections can be painful, more so than collagen injections and most patients require a local anesthetic or numbing agent at the injection site. It takes up to three sessions to achieve the desired effect in most cases. Dermalogen needs to be kept refrigerated. Although it is a natural, human substance, there is still the possibility of an allergic reaction. The visual improvements are short-lived and require multiple treatments. The treatments can be expensive.

## ◈ RADIESSE

Radiesse is a subdermal injectable used to reduce lines and wrinkles and nasolabial folds, and to assist with other skin issues such as scarring and re-contouring. Radiesse treatments are performed in a dermatologist or plastic surgeon's office. Radiesse contains microspheres of calcium hydroxylapatite that are made into a gel that is injected into the desired area. These substances are found naturally in the human body. The gel that is injected into the skin is made up of carbon, sterile water, oxygen, hydrogen and glycerin. Radiesse is injected under the dermis and subcutis layers.

## Advantages of Radiesse

The positive, wrinkle-reducing effects of Radiesse last up to two years. This long-lasting dermal filler greatly diminishes moderate to severe wrinkles and folds in the skin. It is also very effective when used to increase cheek volume, lift jowls, and plump lips. No skin test is required.

Patients can resume normal activities immediately after treatment.

## Disadvantages of Radiesse

Anyone with a history of severe allergies, especially with anaphylactic reactions, may be allergic to Radiesse. Some people exhibit a hypersensitivity to some of the components used. There may be swelling at the injection site, but it usually subsides within 24 to 36 hours. There may be discomfort that can be relieved with medication, and some bruising also occur. Patients should avoid the sun after treatment.

There are some risks of complications following Radiesse injections. Patients may develop nodules that require steroids or surgery to correct. There is also a risk of pain that is resistant to medication. Let your physician know if you experience any abnormal pain. Work with a physician experienced with the use of Radiesse to minimize adverse effects. Radiesse treatments range from $650-$800 for each injection.

## Skin Tightening

With aging comes a sagging skin that makes some people look tired and older than they are. Non–invasive laser procedures can be used to tighten skin and reduce wrinkles with few side effects and little or no down time. Some of the most common skin tightening procedures will be discussed on the next few pages.

### ◈ FRAXEL

Fraxel laser resurfacing is useful for treating wrinkles, crow's feet, facial lines, enlarged pores, age spots, sun spots, scars, melasma, stretch marks, and sun damaged skin. Fraxel results are gradual, and it can take weeks for the full effect to appear. This treatment spares patients extended recovery and downtime. Fraxel can be combined with chemical peels, microdermabrasion, and other laser resurfacing.

Fraxel treatments actually injure microscopic areas of the skin in order to cause the surrounding normal skin to create new tissue. The new skin is tighter and healthier which helps to reduce and minimize any imperfections in the patient's skin. The treatment sessions begin with a thorough skin cleansing. An hour prior to treatment, a topical agent is used to numb the target area. The resurfacing procedure takes 10–25 minutes. Usually, it takes three to five sessions to establish an effective treatment regimen. Fraxel treatments can be done right in the physician's office. Patients generally experience little downtime after treatment, and side effects are usually limited to a few days of redness and swelling followed by some skin exfoliation.

## Advantages of Fraxel

Fraxel offers patients immediate, predictable, positive results every time. Laser technology is precise and accurate, achieving expected results in the targeted areas. Because of the precise nature of the laser, healthy tissue is not harmed, making Fraxel an effective tool for use on thin skin areas such as the neck, face, hands and chest. In most cases, pain is minimal and managed with a topical anesthesia. Compared to more traditional, ablative laser treatments, Fraxel requires fewer treatment sessions to be effective. Most patients are back to normal within seven to ten days.

## Disadvantages of Fraxel

After treatment, patients may experience a mild, sunburned feeling with a pink to red skin tone for about seven days. Your skin will exfoliate (flake off) as new skin replaces dead tissue. You may want to use a moisturizer during the healing process; use a product that you might use for a sun burn to ease the discomfort. A sun block should be used for several months after treatment, and you should avoid direct sunlight. Fraxel treatments cost between $750 and $1,000 per treatment session.

### ◈ PELLEVE

Pelleve was approved by the U.S. Federal Drug Administration in 2009. It is delivered using a laser instrument that provides maximum control in precision cutting and heat delivery. It is used mostly on facial skin such as the corners of eyelids (crow's feet), lines around the mouth and nose, and on moderate to severe wrinkles. Dermatologists, plastic surgeons and other medical professionals should be consulted when considering Pelleve.

With the use of advanced radio frequency technology, Pelleve produces heat by emitting electromagnetic waves into the deep layers of the dermal tissue. This heat breaks down the collagen in the area. When this happens, new collagen forms and the older collagen gets tighter and, in turn, smoothes the outer skin without causing visible skin damage like might be caused by sunburn or skin cancers.

The procedure used during a treatment with Pelleve is non-invasive and virtually painless.

Treatments take between forty-five minutes to an hour to complete; there are no incisions or anesthetics administered. Pelleve can also be used to tighten the skin before a Botox treatment.

## Advantages of Pelleve

The positive effects of Pelleve can last a full six months, with treatment being relatively quick and devoid of pain. There are no permanent side effects with Pelleve, and downtime after the procedure is minimal. Pelleve is a safe option for people seeking a more youthful appearance.

## Disadvantages of Pelleve

Mild, localized discomfort or pain may occur in the treated areas. There may also be some swelling or redness in the area, which will dissipate within twenty-four hours or less. A single Pelleve procedure is about $750 per area. If sagging is expansive or multiple areas need treatment, costs can increase to more than $1500 per area.

## ❖ THERMAGE

Thermage is a device used to tighten the skin, especially in the jowl, neck and eyelid areas. It is a noninvasive tool used to achieve a facelift-like appearance without the need for surgery.

Thermage can help alleviate cellulite, especially in women, tighten the abdominal area, firm upper arm skin that has become loosened with age, tighten sagging buttocks, and address other areas that need strengthening such as breasts and thighs. Thermage uses mono-polar radio frequency energy to heat the underlying skin and remodal deep, dermal collagen to tighten the skin. Thermage works best before the skin becomes too lax with age, so it should be done early.

Thermage treatments take thirty minutes to two hours to administer, depending on the number and size of areas to be treated. If performed in a doctor's office, a light oral sedative can be used to minimize discomfort or feelings of excessive heat. As with most outpatient skin tightening techniques, a board certified dermatologist should be consulted. These treatments have been approved by the Federal Drug Administration.

Thermage can be safely used in conjunction with other types of skin renewal, such as chemical peels, dermal fillers like Botox, Restylane, and Radiesse, and laser therapy.

## Advantages of Thermage

Thermage is a safe alternative to surgical interventions, such as facelifts. Patients can return to normal, everyday activities with no down time. The results of Thermage continue to improve for up to six months, making additional treatments unnecessary.

## Disadvantages of Thermage

Patients may experience mild to moderate swelling and/or redness on the skin. Sunscreen must be worn on the treated areas to protect the skin and prolong the desired results. When large areas of the body are treated, it may take more than one visit to achieve the desired effects.

## ◆ Titan

Undergoing a Titan laser procedure can tighten loose, sagging skin and fix wrinkles by stimulating new collagen production. It is similar to Pelleve and Fraxel in that it is a non-invasive, infrared technology.

Besides its use on facial skin, Titan can also tighten abdominal skin, the skin around the knees, the arms, inner thighs and along the jaw line. Titan uses infrared light to heat an area of collagen just under the skin's surface. It denatures the collagen, but turns cool on the skin's outer surface in order to avoid damage that would be visible to the eye.

A thin layer of gel is smoothed onto the skin's surface during the procedure. to facilitate the movement of the laser, which is passed over the target area. The laser heats the underlying dermal layer, causing the collagen to contract and tighten which then smoothes and refreshes the outer layer of skin. Titan can be used in conjunction with Botox injections for further enhancement. It may take up to six Titan treatments to achieve desired results; treatments are given one month apart.

## Advantages of Titan

Patients can return to normal activities with a minimum of downtime. There is little or no pain associated with Titan treatments, and they are generally safe and well-tolerated. Titan is a progressive collagen builder, and visible results can be seen within a few weeks. Titan can be used on any color skin without negative effects.

## Disadvantages of Titan

Titan is not effective if there is too much loose skin or fat present in the area already. There is a small risk of infection and/or scarring. Studies have shown that only about one-third of Titan patients see dramatic results, and it is very difficult to identify good candidates for this procedure in advance.

## ◈ Photo Rejuvenation

Recent breakthroughs in laser technology and photo rejuvenation have made it possible to erase years off your age without costly and invasive surgical procedures and with little to no downtime.

Photo rejuvenation using IPL represents a breakthrough in age-defying skincare. Photo rejuvenation IPL skin treatments are safe, effective, and a popular way to improve the signs of aging on the face, neck, chest, arms, and hands. This is an office procedure that must be performed by a physician or trained medical staff member. The treatments typically require four to six sessions of about 20 minutes each, performed at three to four week intervals. Photo rejuvenation technology provides dramatic results for a variety of benign conditions, including age spots, sun-induced circles, rosacea, birthmarks, unsightly veins, acne scarring, and other blemishes. Photo rejuvenation skin treatments can be used in conjunction with Botox, Restylane, and microdermabrasion.

Photo rejuvenation is slowly and gradually reducing the number of facelifts that are performed because facelifts and other surgical procedures are too invasive for younger patients and baby boomers who simply want to revitalize their appearances. Photo rejuvenation can be used in conjunction with some medications to treat acne in teenagers and adults.

## ❖ Spider Vein Removal with Lasers

Spider veins are tiny, visible veins just under the surface of the skin. They are different from varicose veins, which are swollen, often painful, and can be surgically removed because they no longer function.

Spider veins can be treated with laser therapy, which is fast and safe. Sclerotherapy is another method used for eliminating spider veins through injections into the veins, but it can take more than five treatments before any results are realized and is often disappointing because the spider veins never go away completely. Laser therapy for spider vein removal, on the other hand, is non-invasive and usually takes only three treatments.

A laser delivers pulses of energy to the surface of the skin, causing the blood within to coagulate; when this happens, the veins shrink and then get reabsorbed by the body. The most advanced laser for spider vein removal is the Nd: YAG laser. It is the laser used most often at medical spas staffed by medical professionals. Laser therapy is the best option for spider veins that have been resistant to sclerotherapy.

Before laser therapy is performed, a doctor must evaluate the patient to make sure there are no underlying problems that may be causing the spider veins.

Most patients do not experience any lasting side effects from the laser, but they may feel a slight burning sensation during the laser therapy. After spider vein laser therapy, patients are required to wear Ace bandages or support hose for a week to ten days. Patients must also avoid hot baths for a few days after treatment and should not participate in any vigorous exercise. Spider veins usually begin to fade a few days after the initial treatment and will continue to improve with additional treatments. Because new spider veins may appear over time, additional laser treatments may be required.

## ◈ MICRODERMABRASION

Microdermabrasion is a non-invasive exfoliating procedure performed individually or in a series to revitalize and maintain the skin's appearance and smoothness. It can be used to address problem areas on the face or body. One session generally takes 30-50 minutes. There is no special preparation required before a procedure, and there is no recuperation needed after.

Microdermabrasion is effective at:

❖ Improving dull or uneven skin color

❖ Eliminating clogged pores and blackheads

❖ Softening general roughness or thickened patches of dead skin (e.g., elbows, feet)

❖ Refining the appearance of fine lines, large pores, acne, and hyperpigmentation

❖ Removing surface debris and allowing the skin to better absorb topical medications

❖ Increasing circulation for a natural glow

❖ The overall youthful appearance of their skin

The procedure may cause slight redness to the skin, but this will subside within a few hours. Although uncommon, some patients may experience blushing of the skin from increased blood flow, but that will fade within a couple of days.

## ◈ How Facials Peels Add Youth and Vibrancy to the Skin

A peel gives your skin a thorough exfoliating treatment, removing dead, dry skin cells on the skin's surface and leaving smoother, softer skin underneath. Learn about the basics of both home and professional peels so you can determine if this treatment is right for you.

### Professional Peels

Professional peels range from superficial peels that require no anesthesia and little recovery time to deep peels that remove significantly more skin and require anesthesia to complete. The type of peel you choose will depend on the results you want to see and the level of damage that has already been done to your skin.

One of the most popular professional peels available today is the PCA peel, which uses alpha hydroxy acids and a variety of other ingredients to address different skin conditions. They are commonly used to treat cystic acne, sun damage, pigment discolorations, and the effects of aging. Most PCA peels do not require any type of anesthesia, although a sedative may be administered for the comfort of the patient. There is little discomfort during or recovery time after the procedure.

## Home Peels

For those who prefer frequent exfoliation in the comfort of their homes, cosmetic peels are available over the counter. Home peels generally use alpha or beta hydroxy acids or a combination of the two. Enzymes may also be used to smooth and clarify the complexion. These peels can be used more frequently and cost much less than professional peels. However, results are not as dramatic, and the treatment will need to be repeated more frequently to achieve desired results.

Elemis offers a papaya enzyme peel that can be used daily to smooth and clarify the skin. This home peel is appropriate for all skin types, including sensitive skin. When the Elemis product is used regularly, it makes a difference in the overall look of the skin without drying the complexion or causing irritation. This product is designed to work best with other Elemis formulas, including the resurfacing facial wash and rejuvenating mask.

PCA Advanced Skincare offers excellent treatment options to rejuvenate and sooth your skin after a peel.

Peels are an excellent way to recharge the skin and eliminate flaws like rough patches, pigmentation irregularities and the effects of aging. The depth of the peel determines how dramatic the results of your treatment will be. Whether you choose a professional peel at the office of a dermatologist or opt for a home skincare system, a peel creates softer, smoother skin.

## ❖ LASER HAIR REMOVAL

Laser hair removal is another non-invasive cosmetic procedure. It is safe and effective for the removal of unwanted hair. Lasers have their greatest impact on hair in the active growth phase. Since individual hairs grow at varying speeds, four to five treatments are needed to remove unwanted hair. Although laser treatments can cause some discomfort, most patients tolerate the procedure well. Some parts of the body are more sensitive than others, so a topical anesthesia may occasionally be necessary. Side effects, if any, are minor. The majority of laser hair removal procedures are performed at medical spas in the United States.

Laser hair removal treatments can have side effects like itching, redness, and swelling, but they will not last for more than three days. In extreme cases, patients may experience burning and hyperpigmentation. In the case of allergic reaction, a physician should be consulted.

## Which Laser Machine to Choose

Lumenis™ LightSheer™ is the most advanced treatment for effective removal of unwanted hair. LightSheer treatments are safe, noninvasive, long-term solutions to unwanted hair on all body parts and on any skin type or complexion. You can resume regular activities immediately following treatments.

## How Does the Area Look After Treatment?

The appearance of the treated area immediately following a procedure will vary from patient to patient depending on the extent of the work and the patient's skin type. Side effects, if any, are minor. They may include redness and swelling around the hair follicle, which is the desired clinical result, and indicates that the follicle has responded to treatment. Most people return to normal activity right away. You will learn about your specific treatments, possible side effects, and the results you can expect during your initial consultation.

## Before Treatment

❖ Do not tweeze, wax, use a depilatory, or undergo electrolysis in the areas you wish to have treated for 6 weeks prior to laser hair removal.

❖ Do not tan the areas to be treated for 4 weeks prior to treatment.

❖ Avoid using self-tanning products for 2 weeks prior to treatment.

❖ Shave the area to be treated prior to your appointment as skin should be free of stubble.

❖ Apply anesthetic cream at least 30 minutes prior to appointment time and cover with plastic wrap.

## After Treatment

❖ Some redness and swelling in the area is normal and may feel similar to sunburn. This sensation should disappear within several hours to several days after treatment.

❖ Gently clean the treated area twice daily.

❖ Avoid irritants (glycolics, retinoids, etc.) for seven days after treatment.

❖ Apply 30 SPF sunscreen daily over the treated area.

❖ Do not use deodorant if underarms are treated.

❖ Avoid exercise until redness has cleared.

❖ Do not pick, scratch, or tweeze the treated area.

❖ Apply 1% hydrocortisone or aloe vera until redness disappears.

❖ Apply ice immediately after treatment if desired.

## How Much Does The Treatment Cost?

The cost of treatment depends on the size of the area being treated, how many treatments are needed, which machine is being used, who performs the procedures, and which technology is being used.

## ❖ HOW TO CHOOSE A MEDICAL SPA FOR YOUR NON –SURGICAL AESTHETIC PROCEDURES

The medical spa business is booming, with more and more clinics that offer non-surgical cosmetic procedures opening up across the country. However, the multitude of options leaves many clients in a quandary, wondering which spa will best meet their needs. Today's savvy consumer needs to be educated in what to look for in a medical spa and the aesthetic procedures it provides to ensure optimal results. This includes evaluating the medical spa and the professionals who work there for experience, credentials, and high safety and success ratings.

As the cosmetic industry booms, clients are unsure which medical spas offer the most effective and safest procedures. A recent report in Aesthetic Medical News showed that clients looking for cosmetic procedures are becoming more adamant about appropriate professional credentials. This trend is expected to continue, according to the research conducted by the International Association for Physicians in Aesthetic Medicine. Jeff Russell, Executive Director of IAPAM, told Aesthetic Medical News, "The results clearly indicate that most women are concerned about their safety when choosing aesthetic procedures."

Short of asking for statistical research, consumers have other avenues to explore when determining the safety of a medical spa and the effectiveness of the procedures it provides. First, find out if the medical spa is truly operated by a doctor. While some spas hire a doctor to work as the 'medical director' of the facility, that medical professional may have no involvement in the daily operations of the spa or even know what type of tools they use for aesthetic procedures. It is critical that the doctor is actively part of the medical spa and its treatments.

Clients can also ask how long the spa has been in business and who, typically, performs the laser hair removal procedures. If an RN does the majority of the treatments, ask what training the nurses have in laser procedures and if a doctor oversees the treatment protocol.

Another important consideration when choosing a medical spa is the type of laser being used. Clients should never opt for a medical spa just because it offers a lower price if that facility is using inferior machines for its treatments – to do so would result in more sessions to achieve desired results, and additional treatments can raise costs significantly in the long run.

# ತ 10 ಜ

# COMPANIES OF NOTE

O ver the past few decades, the skin care industry has grown exponentially. New skin care brands are introduced in the market every day. As an educated consumer, you will want to apply the information you gained from this book when you plan a new skin care regimen or update your existing program. We have reviewed some of the leading brands for you in this chapter.

## ❖ AGELESS DERMA

Ageless Derma was developed by a committed group of physicians, chemists, researchers and estheticians with over 30 years of experience. At the heart of this anti-aging range are high concentration stem cells, peptides and antioxidants that have been drawn from nature to provide flawless skin without resorting to invasive or painful delivery techniques. Its products also contain many botanical ingredients, enhanced by the knowledge and innovation of its expert researchers.

The Ageless Derma line contains 3 core products:

❖ Ageless Derma Stem Cell and Peptide Anti-Wrinkle Cream

❖ Ageless Derma Retinol and Vitamin K Eye Cream

❖ Ageless Derma Anti-Aging Skin brightener

Ageless Derma also offers an all-natural line of anti-aging mineral makeup that is free from all oils and parabens. It contains Vitamin A, E and green tea extract. As natural products contain sensitive ingredients that can be damaged by contact with air and sunlight, Ageless Derma has developed an airless pump to package its products. This process ensures that all of its ingredients remain potent and active, without resorting to the use of harmful preservatives found in other anti-aging ranges.

## ◈ ALYRIA

The Alyria line of products is formulated to improve the skin's tone and texture, to reduce fine lines and wrinkles, and to improve the overall look and radiance of the skin.

The Alyria line of skincare products include:

**Glycolic Acid** — This ingredient is often used to treat rough skin in need of toning and refining. It is also helpful in treating fine lines and hyperpigmentation. Alyria delivers glycolic acid through a patented system called the Amphoteric System. This system controls the release of free acid molecules into the skin while at the same time delivering glycolic acid at its optimum strength.

**Retinol** — Retinol, derived from pure vitamin A, is widely used for fighting wrinkles and refining pores. Through Alyria's patented-release micro-delivery system, Retinol is delivered via Alyria's Retinol Night Complex Level I and Retinol Night Complex Level 2.

**Matrixyl** — Matrixyl, a pentapeptide that helps stimulate collagen synthesis and promotes tissue and wrinkle repair is found in Alyria's Revitalizing Cream and Revitalizing Eye Serum.

**Vitamin K** — Vitamin K is the foundation for Alyria's Anti-Dark Circle Night Serum, which is designed to reduce the appearance of dark circles. Along with vitamin

A, the vitamin K in the Anti-Dark Circle Night Serum is delivered deep into the skin throughout the night.

## ◈ ASTARA

Moving to Telluride, Colorado in 1995 was the realization of a lifelong dream for Sunny Griffin, a former supermodel. However, Griffin quickly realized that the higher altitude and dry climate were wreaking havoc on her skin, causing it to age prematurely. To address these issues, she created and introduced the Astara Natural Skincare line in 1997.

The Astara Natural Skincare line features a wide range of formulas to address every skincare issue. The products are divided into four basic categories: cleansing, repairing, reviving and replenishing. Astara also offers body care products like its Aquatherapy Body Care Collection and Bath Moods Kit. The Blue Flame line is specifically geared to oily skin prone to breakouts, while the antioxidant formulas are packed with nutrients like vitamins A, C and E to fight the environmental free radicals that lead to premature aging.

Many of the Astara formulas offer skincare ingredients found in the sea, including mineral-rich sea salts and seaweed extracts. A great deal of research has been done on the benefits of such ingredients, and Astara ensures that they use only the highest quality marine botanicals and minerals.

Astara Natural Skincare products have been used to cleanse and nurture skin for more than a decade. Products are available through the Astara website, as well as through numerous high end retailers.

## ◈ B. KAMINS

This company has been a pioneer in treating rosacea, sun damage, and the effects of aging. Today, B. Kamins offers a comprehensive product line that targets an extensive range of problems and skin types for both men and women. B. Kamins products are available through high-end spas and online retailers.

B. Kamins Chemist originally began creating skincare formulas for family members more than 40 years ago. The company became "official" in the 1990s, after Howard Kaminsky, the son of chemist Ben Kaminsky, recognized that the formulas his father had designed could be marketed as a unique skincare option for the general public. Howard and his father began working together to create a product that could be sold through spas and eventually directly to the general public through retail centers.

B. Kamins offers three trademark technologies that are used in many of their products:

**Bio-Maple Compound** — Derived from the Canadian Acer Saccharum maple trees, this ingredient has been shown to counter moisture loss in the skin while providing much needed antioxidants and nutrients that protect the skin from the aging process.

**Episphere Blue** — This time-released vitamin E formula helps prevent aging due to its high antioxidant content and moisturizing ability.

**Profusion Ceramide** — This substance plumps skin from the inside out, smoothing fine lines and wrinkles, for a smoother, younger appearance.

## ◈ BABOR

Babor was founded in 1956 by Dr. Michael Babor under the name Dr. Babor GmbH. The first product introduced in the skincare line was a cleanser containing "hydrophilic oil," known today as HY-OL. Today, Babor is one of the leading companies in professional cosmetics and has a presence in more than 60 countries around the world. The products can be purchased through high end retailers or spas, and through the company's website.

Babor uses formulas that are rich in natural oils, like macadamia, soybean, and peanut oil, as well as nutrients like vitamins A, E and C. Some formulas also contain proven hydrating essentials like hyaluronic acid and shea butter.

Babor skincare products are appropriate for nearly any skin type, with some lines that address specific skin issues. Oily skin responds best to the Babor Cleansing Gel and Tonic containing salicylic acid, which keeps pimples at bay, while those with dry skin might consider the Moist Intense Ultra Hydrating Cream with hyaluronic acid and vitamin E and the Vita Balance Lipid Plus with sesame oil. People with mature skin can turn back the clock with products like the Derma Cellular Ultimate Wrinkle Control Fluid with collagen and protein complexes. The Nanocell Age Protecting Cream is designed to prolong the life of skin stem cells for a more youthful complexion.

Babor also offers a full line of body care products, such as Body Line Thermal. In addition to standard shower gels and body creams, the line also features a bust lifting formula and a cellulite treatment.

## ◈ BECCA COSMETICS

The Becca Cosmetics Line, tested for more than six years, was founded by Rebecca Williams. A talented and highly regarded make-up artist, Williams was not satisfied with the cosmetics lines that were currently available.

Williams developed a Three-Step Skin Perfecting Makeup System that addressed women of all ages and races. This make-up is designed to heal while it conceals and works to even out skin tones and restore natural glow.

This line (which is never tested on animals) offers more than thirty different shades of concealers and foundations. Lip, cheek, and eye color/mascara are also important parts of the Becca line, along with moisturizers, bronzers, glitters and primers.

## ◈ Bioelements

Bioelements was founded by Barbara Salomone, one of the first licensed aestheticians in the United States. Salomone's goal was to create a line of products that could address specific skin issues, like acne and aging, and transform the way professionals treat the skin. With the help of a team of cosmetic chemists and expert aestheticians, the Bioelements line was born..

Bioelements offers formulas for all skin types, so treatments can address the user's specific needs. Custom blending is available to aestheticians who can pinpoint the ingredients your skin needs in the right proportions to achieve optimum results. For home use, products are available for oily, dry and aging skin, as well as for target areas like the eyes and lips, sun-damaged skin, and sensitive skin. The company also offers a skincare line for men.

## ◈ Borba Skincare

Borba was founded by Scott-Vincent Borba, who was unable to find skincare products that could help him effectively heal his blemished skin. Borba Skincare uses two formulas—one is ingestible, while the other is topical. The products are also nutraceutical (a combination of nutrition and pharmaceuticals) and cosmaceuticals (a combination of cosmetics and pharmaceuticals) and are available as creams, lotions, cleansers, and other products to attack blemishes and wrinkles.

## ◈ CLAYTON SHAGAL

Clayton Shagal was started in 1982 in Quebec, where it produced and sold one collagen gel product. Now, Clayton Shagal has a complete skincare line that is focused on fighting the signs of aging by offering products for both men and women. Clayton Shagal products are designed to be simple, natural, and effective. It develops its skincare products around elastin, water, and collagen, which are the basic components of the skin.

Clayton Shagal uses only 7 active ingredients in its product line: proteoglycans, cytokines, collagen (to help aging skin look more youthful), elastin (to increase firmness), hydrocomplex (to encourage moisture retention), placenta (with its healing effect) and hynoderm (which keeps moisture in the skin).

Clayton Shagal products are designed for every skin type and are effective for promoting youthful skin in men and women. Clayton Shagal Colhy Gel stimulates new collagen production, which, in turn, helps smooth and prevent fine lines and wrinkles from appearing. Clayton Shagal Colhy Gel also tightens pores and gives the skin a smoother, firmer look. The line features Collagen Gel for sensitive skin, acne, rosacea, broken capillaries, and couperose.

## ◈ CLIENTELE

Using unusual ingredients such as pumpkin, extract of Lotus seeds, flowers and Estrokin, and powerful antioxidants, Clientele's products help slow your skin's aging process.

The Elastology line provides cleansers, body care, age erasers, exfoliators, nourishing skin serums, and anti wrinkle creams.

Estro-lift offers seven different types of firming and nourishing serums, including their Intensive Serum, which plumps and regenerates skin to restore the supple look of youth.

## ◈ CLINICIANS COMPLEX SKINCARE

Clinicians Complex, formerly known as Physicians Complex, is a family of anti-aging skincare products designed to penetrate the surface of the skin and infuse it with rich elements. Designed for use on adult skin types, Clinicians Complex is a comprehensive anti-aging skincare system specially formulated to treat the unique chemistry of the skin. Elements of Retinol, glycolic acid, and vitamin C-Ester work in harmony to treat the skin as they nourish and protect it.

The Clinicians Complex product line is ideal for the treatment of common skin concerns such as sun damage, adult acne, and wrinkles. Products are specifically formulated to rejuvenate the skin from the inside, without causing damage or irritation. Clinicians Complex skincare products are available only through medical spas and other establishments directly associated with physicians.

## ◈ COLORESCIENCE

Colorescience offers a wide range of mineral-based skincare and cosmetic products. The formulas in the Colorescience line are devoid of artificial fillers, including talc, dyes and perfumes, which are commonly seen in many cosmetic and skincare products today. The founder of the company, Diane Ranger, was the original inventor of mineral makeup and coined the phrase in 1977. Today,

Ranger has found a way to incorporate minerals into many types of skincare products. Colorescience is available through high end spas and can also be purchased online.

Mineral makeup is a large and growing trend in the cosmetic industry right now, leading some companies to create lower quality products for the sake of turning a profit. Consumers should use caution when shopping for mineral-based cosmetics to ensure the products they select are free of the unhealthy fillers that block the effectiveness of the minerals.

The Colorescience line includes the following:

❖ Skincare products for the face

❖ Formulas specifically designed for the eyes and lips

❖ Sun protection formulas

❖ Post-treatment kits used by spas and professional aestheticians

Colorescience skincare products are broken down to address specific skin issues, including problem skin, sensitive skin, and skin that is prone to redness or discoloration. The skincare lines incorporate cleansers, primers, sun protection, and foundation that can camouflage problems as it treats them. Face enhancement products include a broad spectrum of cosmetics. Many formulas come with sun protection up to SPF 50 to help prevent future damage while it treats current issues.

## ◈ CosMedix

CosMedix offers fourteen products to correct and stimulate your skin, enhancing the skin's natural healing process by supporting external barriers and acting as an anti-inflammatory. Each supplement offers benefits for different needs, such as exfoliating for acne prone skin,

skin lightening for hyper-pigmentation, and antioxidants for aging skin.

CosMedix Correct & Repair products assist the skin's natural healing process. From the Benefit Clean Gentle Cleanser and Phytoclear Clarifying Moisturizer to the Rescue Healing Balm and Mask, these specialty ingredients cover a wide array of common skin conditions, while CosMedix's line of sun protection products deflect potentially harmful ultraviolet radiation. Correct & Protect products provide full spectrum natural UVA/UVB/UVC sun block protection and hydration for all skin types.

CosMedix offers a wide variety of skin peels to correct various skin conditions. These natural peels soothe the skin and stimulate collagen production without the side effects of harsh, damaging chemicals. CosMedix also offers a "physicians only" medical strength L-TCA peel that causes much less discomfort and downtime than traditional TCA peels.

These medical strength formulas correct body-specific skin conditions and compliment patient treatment programs administered by dermatologists and aesthetic physicians.

## ◈ COSMEDERM

The Refinity COSMEDERM-7 Skin Solutions system begins with an in-office peel designed to accelerate exfoliation, followed up with at-home products for maximum results. The office peel is 70% glycolic acid; it diminishes the appearance of fine lines and wrinkles and improves the skin's texture and tone. Unlike typical cosmetic peels, the Refinity COSMEDERM-7 Skin Solutions peel causes little irritation to the skin due to COSMEDERM-7's patented anti-irritant.

COSMEDERM-7 is the commercial name for naturally occurring strontium salt compounds that have been clinically proven to minimize, and even eliminate, much of the skin irritation that accompanies high acid-level facial peels.

It is important to point out that COSMEDERM-7 is not a topical anesthetic and does not numb the face during a procedure; rather, it greatly reduces the sensory irritation by as much as 77%.

COSMEDERM-7 allows the Refinity Skin Solutions peel to deliver the highest concentrations of active ingredients that would otherwise be too irritating on the skin. In other words, effectiveness is maximized and discomfort is minimized during and after a Refinity Skin Solutions peel with COSMEDERM-7.

The Refinity Skin Solutions facial peel is an in-office procedure that takes no more than 30 minutes to complete. The soothing properties of COSMEDERM-7 means individuals experience very little irritation and can resume normal activities almost immediately following treatment.

## ◈ DDF

Dr. Sobel originally founded HDS Cosmetic Lab in 1991, where he produced skincare formulas to use on his own patients. The focus of HDS formulas was to unite cosmetic dermatology with topical skincare for products that provided stellar results without a prescription. Two years later, Dr. Sobel's sister, nutritional expert Elaine Linker, joined the company to help expand production and educate the general public about the products. The company also recruited the expertise of a leading biochemist to explore the field of cell physiology and how it relates to skincare.

In 1995, Dr. Sobel changed the name of his company to DDF - Doctor's Dermatologic Formula. At the same time, the company adopted a skincare philosophy of "cleanse, protect and treat" and today, all of the products in the line are precisely formulated to accommodate these important skincare steps.

DDF uses a variety of ingredients in their formulas, including natural botanicals, marine extracts, and proven anti-aging ingredients like hyaluronic acid and peptides. Acne fighting formulas include substances like glycolic acid and sulfur, while skin brightening products offer additions like hydroquinone.

DDF categorizes products by skin type, making it easy for customers to find the precise formulas that match their needs. The anti-aging products are divided between preventative and restorative care, so you can choose your formulas based on your age and the amount of skin damage you have already experienced. Customers can also shop for products based on the formula purpose, such as cleansers, moisturizers and specific treatments.

DDF provides a number of skincare kits, making it easy for customers to choose the products that work together for best results. The Decelerate Professional Anti-Aging Protocol kit includes a wash containing glycolic acid for gentle exfoliation, a daily moisturizer with an SPF 15 to prevent further sun damage, and a protective cream specifically designed for the eyes. The kit also includes a healthy cell serum that includes potent peptides, amino acids, and antioxidants to correct current signs of aging and prevent future damage from occurring.

## ◈ DERMABLEND

Dermablend does not offer treatment options for problem skin. Instead, this company specializes in camouflage methods that effectively hide imperfections currently being treated or those that don't respond well to treatment.

Dermablend was started in 1981 by Dr. Craig Roberts and his wife Florie. The original intention of the company was to become the premier provider of corrective makeup, and today, Dermablend has achieved that goal.

The Dermablend concealer, like all of the other Dermablend products, is non-comedogenic, non-acnegenic, and free of artificial fragrances. This means that users can be assured that Dermablend products will effectively hide skin conditions without irritating the skin or making the condition worse.

In addition to effective ingredients designed to conceal nearly any skin flaw, Dermablend uses titanium dioxide in many of its formulas to offer sun protection. The Dermablend concealer comes with a standard SPF 30..

Dermablend products address concerns including dark circles, age spots, and freckles. Body concealers are available to hide problems like stretch marks, spider veins and even tattoos. Chronic skin conditions like rosacea can be treated with a Dermablend concealer.

One secret to Dermablend's success is the setting powder that can be used over any Dermablend concealer or foundation. This loose setting powder contains micronized talc that effectively sets makeup and makes it last longer. This powder comes in three shades: original, for all skin tones; cool beige, for medium skin tones; and warm saffron, for deeper skin tones. Dermablend leg and body cover is also designed to be used in combination to minimize the appearance of skin conditions like spider veins.

## ◈ DERMALOGICA

Dermalogica brings more than 25 years of experience to the table. It was created by The International Dermal Institute, which was founded by British skin-care therapist Jane Wurwand in 1983, when she discovered a need to educate and train aestheticians in the United States. Wurwand began with a single, small classroom in Marina

Del Rey, California; today, IDI offers world class skincare training in more than 40 locations worldwide.

The Dermalogica skincare formulas improve skin health without harsh ingredients that might irritate the skin. Dermalogica substitutes many of the common synthetic ingredients found in skincare formulas today with natural botanicals and proven substances to treat a host of skin concerns.

While Dermalogica products claim to be gentle enough for any skin type, product systems are also broken into categories to address very specific skin concerns. The MediBac line is designed for people dealing with adult acne, while the UltraCalming Line is recommended for people with sensitive skin. Aging skin responds best to the AGE Smart skincare line that comes complete with cleansers, moisturizers, and treatment options that can turn back time and prevent future damage. The Daylight Defense products provide potent SPF protection while offering the skin essential nutrients at the same time. Dermalogica also offers formulas to treat sun damage by soothing and repairing burned skin. The company's line of skin brighteners offers formulas with peptides and other ingredients that work together to even skin tone and produce a brighter, younger looking complexion.

## ◈ DermaNew

DermaNew is the brainchild of Beverly Hills salon owners Amby Longhofer and Dean Rhoades. Their goal was to bring the best office and spa treatments into the home in a safe, easy, and affordable manner. This led them to discover new methods for microdermabrasion that users could apply in the privacy and comfort of their own homes. Their philosophy is, "Don't settle for anything less than the best. Use only what the pros of Beverly Hills would use."

DermaNew offers a complete microdermabrasion system in many unique formulas, including moisturizers, mousses, gels, masques, foams, creams, sun protectors, cleansers, body washes, serums, bleaches, lighteners, and exfoliants. These products can accomplish a great number of things and are suitable for all skin types—sensitive, dry, oily, a combination of these, or normal. There are also formulas created specifically for acne and excessive oil. The company offers products designed for the whole body, the face, the eyes, the feet, and the hands and nails. There are products that can be used during the day or overnight, and the line also includes tools (e.g., for callous softening) and kits containing a cross-section of several products.

Corundum is the primary ingredient in DermaNew, but the line has also included a handful of other natural and pure components, like green tea, and carrot and grape seed extracts. You will see improvements as soon as one week after treatment begins, including less clogged pores, more even skin tone and pigmentation, and significantly fewer blackheads. As DermaNew cures these problems by removing the first layer of skin, it also helps to improve scars and wrinkles.

### ❖ DERMAQUEST

Sam Dhatt started Dermaquest Skin Therapy in 1999 with the goal of developing skincare products using the latest scientific developments and ingredients. Mr. Dhatt is a renowned cosmaceutical chemist and is also CEO of a manufacturing company. He is among the first to learn about new skincare ingredients, which he then tests extensively in his own laboratory before putting them on the market. Dermaquest Skin Therapy exercises complete control over every stage of the development process, from initial ideas and testing to production and distribution.

Dermaquest Skin Therapy products utilize ingredients like alpha lipoic acid, hydrating hyaluronic acid, MDI complex, and antioxidant co-enzyme Q10. Hyaluronic Acid (HA) is found in the connective tissues of humans. HA promotes skin hydration because it is able to hold 1,000 times its molecular weight in moisture. This results in hydrated skin that is smoother and more supple. Dermaquest also uses a MDI complex that is made up of extracted fish cartilage. This MDI complex prevents the breakdown of the skin's collagen and also improves hydration and skin firmness while reducing dark circles and redness from broken capillaries and UV damage. The co-enzyme Q10 increases healthy cell renewal.

The Peptide Mobilizer helps skin thicken by stimulating collagen, glycosaminoglycans, and fibronectin. It also keeps skin hydrated, reduces muscle contractions that cause wrinkles, and promotes skin cell regeneration. Peptide Mobilizer also increases the positive effects from skin treatments like peels and resurfacers.

Another Dermaquest product is ZinClear, a sunscreen with zinc oxide that won't leave telltale white residue on the skin. ZinClear is for normal and sensitive skin, and with its broad spectrum coverage, will help prevent sun damage caused by exposure to UVB and UVA rays.

## ❖ Dr. Brandt

Dr. Brandt brings more than 20 years of experience as a dermatologist to his skincare line. He is a board certified member of the American Board of Internal Medicine and the American Board of Dermatology. In addition to creating his skincare line, Dr. Brandt is known for his educational contributions to the field of skincare and dermatology, his numerous research programs, and his professional papers and manuals.

The philosophy behind the Dr. Brandt's skincare line is to offer high quality, potent formulas with results similar to those you might expect from a visit to the dermatologist. Products are packed with high quality botanicals and scientifically proven ingredients designed to effectively address a host of skin concerns. Today, customers can find Dr. Brandt skincare products through online retailers, as well as numerous brick and mortar stores across the country.

Dr. Brandt products combine natural ingredients with scientifically proven substances to address a wide range of skin concerns. Acne fighting formulas incorporate traditional ingredients like salicylic acid with a host of soothing botanicals and scientifically proven peptides.

One of Dr. Brandt's newest skincare lines is the Time Arrest line that offers potent anti-aging ingredients like peptides and phospholipids.

Dr. Brandt breaks down products by skin type, allowing customers to find the best formulas for their needs quickly and easily. Blemishes No More is a skincare line specifically for oily skin, with acne-fighting ingredients like salicylic acid and soothing botanicals to reduce redness and inflammation. Pores No More is another option for oily skin, with alpha and beta hydroxy acids that pack a powerful punch against enlarged pores and blackheads. Dr. Brandt's House Calls products claim to mimic the effects of a professional treatment right in your home, and the company's microdermabrasion products are particularly popular, with both lactic and glycolic acid to help slough off dead, dry skin cells and leave a healthy glow behind.

## ◈ DR. DENNIS GROSS

Dr. Dennis Gross Skincare is named for the Manhattan dermatologist who designed the line. Dr. Gross has devoted his professional life to the study of skin health and the reversal of sun damage. Dr. Gross has established himself as one of the premiere dermatologists and experts on skincare in the country.

The Dr. Dennis Gross skincare line was originally introduced to the market in 2002 as MD Skincare, with a string of multi-purpose products designed to create a more beautiful complexion.

The Dr. Dennis Gross line includes a variety of cleansers, moisturizers, and peels for every skin type and need. It includes an extensive line of sun protection formulas and body care products. Some of their other popular lines include the Alpha Beta and Hydra Pure products.

The biggest seller in the Dr. Dennis Gross skincare line is the Alpha Beta daily face peel, a two-step system for gently exfoliating the skin every day. The peel can be combined with products from the Hydra Pure line, such as the Firming Serum and Vitamin C Brightening Serum, for improved results.

The Dr. Dennis Gross line may be a relative newcomer to skincare products, but it has quickly gained popularity as one of the top high-end lines in the industry. These formulas work well on all types of skin, nourishing as they treat for a potent result without a prescription.

## ❖ ELEMIS

This product line is varied, and each product is specially formulated to address concerns for each skin type, skin condition and even gender. Although all of the Elemis products are cross gender effective, there are products that are also specially formulated for men to address some of their concerns such as shaving. The company offers an Energizing Skin Scrub containing Hops and Laurel that, when used weekly, can prevent ingrown hairs caused by shaving.

Elemis products are formulated to prevent the effects of aging. Its Pro-Collagen Marine Cream is a global best seller designed to help boost production of facial collagen. This product has been tested in a clinical trial setting where patients saw a reduction of wrinkle depth of up to 78% in just two weeks.

## ❖ EMINENCE

Eminence formulas combat the effects that environmental free radicals, from the sun's ultraviolet rays, smoke, and pollution, ultimately contribute to the signs of aging and even to certain types of diseases. By taking advantage of the fruit pulp, seeds, and peels, this line has been able to design fresh, environmentally-friendly products for your skin.

We all know by now that most of the human body is comprised of water, and it is in constant need of replenishment. Eminence products utilize thermal water, which comes from hot spring lakes in Hungary and provides natural mineral salts as well as a healthy pH balance. This is one of the reasons that the Eminence products are suitable for every skin type, whether it be oily, dry, sensitive, or a combination. Before it is used, the water is fermented and heated, maximizing its potency and abilities.

## ❖ EXUVIANCE

The Exuviance line was developed from the vigorous study of Alpha Hydroxy, Poly Hydroxy, and Bionic Poly Hydroxy Acids. It offers unique blends of these acids, combined with other beneficial skin ingredients such as vitamins A, C, and E.

The Exuviance product line ranges in offerings, from the Acne-Prone Collection that addresses the needs of individuals affected by acne, to products like the Moisture Balance Toner made specifically for dry skin, to the Vespera Bionic Serum.

## ◈ G.M. COLLIN

G.M. Collin was founded in France by a renowned, experienced aesthetician and dermatologist who pioneered the use of collagen in anti-aging products. GM Collin has become known for using the latest technology to develop innovative skincare products. G.M. Collin skincare products are formulated with natural plant and marine extracts and are designed to achieve visible results in a way that supports and assists natural skin minerals. Products are not tested on animals, demonstrating the company's respect for the environment in designing its skincare products.

The GM Collin Exfoliating Gel is formulated with organic green tea and ginger extracts. Its 2 in 1 formula exfoliates and cleanses, refining the skin's texture. It contains polyethylene microspheres that remove dead skin cells without causing irritation. This exfoliating and cleansing gel leaves the skin feeling fresh, hydrated and soft, and it helps optimize the effect of subsequent body care products.

The G.M. Collin H50 Therapy Serumis has been specifically formulated for women experiencing hormonal changes before, during, and after menopause. It combines natural ingredients such as Padina Pavonica and Iris Florentina with five targeted peptides, including Collaxyl and Matrixyl™ 3000. This G.M. Collin H50 therapy serum rebalances the skin's optimal cellular activity and counters the visible signs of hormonal, chronological, and environmental aging, while reducing the appearance of fine lines and deep wrinkles.

## ◈ GLOMINERALS

Glominerals was originally launched in 1998 by Bare Minerals. At that time, mineral-based cosmetics were just coming into vogue, with a number of companies cashing in on the mineral craze. However, the market also saw its share of less-than-stellar products containing synthetic fillers and other substances that interfered with the benefits the minerals were supposed to provide. Glominerals countered the lower-quality products by providing pharmaceutical grade ingredients, potent antioxidants, and triple-milled minerals for cosmetics that would protect and treat the skin. An antioxidant complex containing vitamins A, C and E, and green tea extract protect the skin from environmental free radical damage and ward off the signs of aging. "Triple-milled" ensures that the minerals go into the formulas in their purest form for excellent coverage without causing skin irritation.

Glominerals offers a wide range of cosmetics for the face, eyes and lips. They also have an extensive selection of base products that include foundations and concealers. Eye shadows come in individual, triple, and quad offerings to mix and match as you like, or simply choose the pre-packaged set that you like best.

Lip color is available in traditional lipstick, gloss, or a lip plumping formula that produces a sexy pout made with marine extracts. Lip pencils help keep color in place, while gloTint for cheeks and lips makes it easy to coordinate your look with a single product. Foundations and concealers are rich in antioxidants and UV protection so your skin remains healthy while blemishes and discolorations remain discretely under wraps. Customers can choose between powder and liquid applications, depending on their skin type and individual needs.

## ◈ GlyMed

GlyMed is the brainchild of master medical esthetician, Christine Heathman, who has worked in the skincare industry for more than 25 years. She has made it her life's work to understand the relationship between the skin and the ingredients that we put on it.

GlyMed Plus was the first skincare line to pioneer comprehensive skin color identification, and Christine has become an expert in nearly all cosmetic modalities. As a result, GlyMed has become a world leader in skincare and is the first choice for many skincare and medical professionals around the globe.

Some of the skincare products in the GlyMed Plus line include:

❖ Age Management Skincare System

❖ Serious Action Acne Management

❖ Cell Science

❖ GlyMed Plus Facial Hydrator—a lightweight moisturizing hydrator that accelerates cell renewal and decreases the appearance of fine lines and wrinkles

❖ GlyMed PLUS Treatment Cream with 15 percent Glycolic Acid – helps repair the skin while reducing the appearance of fine lines and wrinkles overnight

❖ GlyMed PLUS AHA Accelerator- a lightweight serum that works with the skin's natural immune system.

## ◈ Glytone

Glytone was originally created by two pharmacists who were some of the first to explore the benefits of glycolic acid to the skin. After many years of study, Genesis Pharmaceuticals was created in 1992 to market the glycolic acid-based skincare products known as the Glytone line. Ten years later, Pierre Fabre Dermo-Cosmetique purchased Genesis Pharmaceuticals and the Glytone brand, providing the brand with its more than 45 years experience in the pharmaceutical industry. Today, Glytone is the only American brand sold by Pierre Fabre Dermo-Cosmetique.

Glycolic acid has long been thought to be the best alpha hydroxy acid available for effective penetration of the skin. Glytone products use a free form glycolic acid that provides a greater benefit to the skin than the more primitive form of the substance.

In addition to glycolic acid, Glytone products also include a wealth of other nutrient-rich ingredients that treat the skin to a healthy, glowing complexion, such as a combination of antioxidants that protect the skin from environmental free radical damage that can lead to early aging. The Glytone antioxidant regimen is primarily designed for anti-aging through the use of the serum, cream, and eye cream that are included in the collection. Glytone also offers clients with acne-prone skin a set of products with both glycolic and salicylic acids to keep breakouts at bay.

## ◈ Guinot

Guinot features a wide range of beauty products that address the needs of both men and women of nearly any age and with any skin type.

One of the main focuses of the Guinot line of skin and body care products is the effect that environmental conditions and stress have on an individual's skin. Keeping those factors in mind, Guinot developed an array of products that protect and moisturize during the day while they strengthen skin tissues and increases circulation and cellular activity during the night.

All Guinot products are designed to work together through an exclusive method.

## ◈ JUARA

The natural skincare line Juara is similar to many other product lines. It has products that are specifically formulated to address specific skin types. It also encourages clients to focus on skincare rituals that are part of the Indonesian tradition that served as the company's inspiration.

Juara products are sold as "mini-ritual" sets. These sets provide everything you need to perform your own skincare rituals. A sample of a basic ritual set would be the Back to Basics 3-Step Set. This kit includes a cleanser, toner, and moisturizer.

Because Juara uses ingredients that are localized to the region, rice and tea may play a more prominent role in the Juara natural skincare line than they might in those of some of its close competitors.

In addition to these products, Juara also has a line of products to address the more common skin problems that we all experience. They have treatments for sensitive skin, repair lotions for sun damage and aging, and acne specific products to help treat breakouts. In addition to the products designed for facial care, they also have lip care products. These include the Sweet Black Tea lip treatment and Candlenut Lip Balm. Shower scrubs and specialty products, like facial masks, round out the Juara offerings.

## ◈ JURLIQUE

Jurlique has a wide product range that includes an organic skincare line, but which also includes bath products, aromatherapy, hair, and baby focused products. The unique thing about this Australian company is that it is in control of every aspect of its product creation process. Instead of sourcing ingredients, it owns a farming operation that produces the key ingredients for the product lines.

Jurlique includes some ingredients in the organic skincare line that are prized for their skincare properties such as lavender and rose, but it also uses some more unique, organic ingredients, such as Ibisabolbol and Turmeric extract. Ibisabolbol helps reduce redness, and turmeric destroys free radicals before they can damage the skin.

Jurlique's product line is incredibly diverse, so most people will be able to find products that meet their needs. Its skincare line includes products that are designed for specific skin types and specific purposes. Gift sets are available for purchase, and they include all the products needed to address specific concerns. Examples include the Rebalance Dryness Introductory Set and the Rebalance Sensitivity Introductory Set.

Products combine primary ingredients from the line with other ingredients that target specific problems. For example, one of the most popular products in the lineup is the Purely Age-Defying Facial Serum. This is an anti-aging product that makes the skin stronger and more elastic. In addition to some of the company's primary ingredients, it also includes Hibiscus, Black Elder, and licorice.

## ◈ KINERASE SKINCARE

The Kinerase Skincare range is built around kinetin, a substance found in plants that prevents them from drying out, withering, and wrinkling. The brand includes creams formulated for day use that can be used in conjunction with make-up, as well as creams intended specifically for night use only. Many of the Kinerase formulas also have SPF built in.

All of the Kinerase formulas are infused with rich botanicals and powerful age-fighting ingredients, such as kola nut, lemon, and aloe vera, as well as more traditional ingredients like salicylic acid, glycolic acid, and hyaluronic acid.

## ◈ LA ROCHE POSAY

Before La Roche Posay became the largest spa resort in Europe and the founder of a popular skincare line, it was a well known French village that dated back to the 12th century. People in the village discovered that the natural thermal waters provided therapeutic healing to a host of skin problems. Today, the spa hosts about 10,000 visitors every year. These people come to take part in treatments for stubborn skin conditions like rosacea, psoriasis, and eczema.

These waters are rich in important minerals like selenium, calcium, and magnesium, and offer a wide range of skin benefits to those who visit. Today, that therapeutic quality is found in La Roche Posay's home skincare products, which combine the healing waters with scientific innovation for results-based skincare formulas. La Roche Posay is now a part of L'Oreal, where development continues as scientists seek to find the best possible skincare options for every skin type and need.

Although the benefits in the waters used by La Roche Posay were discovered in the 16th century, the company became a household name in 1989 when they merged with the L'Oreal group. The village's therapeutic thermal waters form the base for most of the La Roche Posay skincare products, but the water is combined with a range of other selected ingredients for optimal results.

This company was responsible for introducing Madecassoside to the anti-aging skincare market in 2003. Madecassoside offers regenerative functions to dermal structure in order to effectively turn back the clock on the skin. In addition, this company widely uses active C in its formulas to treat skin conditions, because of its ability to restore healthy skin and promote healing.

The La Roche Posay line is an extensive one. Mela-D Serum is one of the top La Roche Posay sellers; it can correct hyperpigmentation and make the skin tone more even. Ingredients like glycolic acid, LHA and Kojic acid make this formula particularly effective. The Active C Eyes formula uses active and stable L-ascorbic acid to diminish the appearance of fine lines, wrinkles, and dark circles.

In addition to the basic La Roche Posay line, the company also offers the Anthelios line, which is specifically geared to offer sun protection. Anthelios produces a variety of sun care products, including daily care, children's formulas, and products specifically designed for outdoor days. Anthelios is considered one of the top options in UVA protection, with advanced, patented sunscreen technologies that prevent sun damage and age-related symptoms.

## ◈ LIERAC

Lierac Paris was started in 1975 by Dr. Leon Cariel, a brilliant physician who combined the proven powers of botanical ingredients with highly-developed, advanced scientific technology. Lierac Laboratories was later bought by Patrick Alès, the man who founded the botanical hair care line Phyto. Lierac products address specific skin issues that occur on the face and body using a host of healthy ingredients, such as ivy, alchemilla, horsetail extracts, active caffeine, arnica, alfalfa, terminalia, among others.

The company offers lotions, exfoliants, creams, eye make-up removers, gels, foaming gels, shaving foams, aftershave moisturizers and gels, and serums.

## ◈ Luzern

When substances are classified as "pharmaceutical grade", it means they use a higher level of active ingredients than products you typically purchase over the counter. These ingredients pack a powerful punch in fighting the effects of aging and maintaining a healthy glow on the skin throughout life. Ingredients used by Luzern, like coQ10 and vitamin C, at this dosage can offer the greatest benefit to the skin with eight times the average active ingredients of other brands.

Luzern uses plants grown in a harsh alpine climate. As a result, these plants tend to have a higher concentration of nutrients, like antioxidants that fight the effects of free radicals in the environment that lead to aging skin. The Bio-Swiss harvesting and extraction process used to remove these substances from the plants and place them into the skincare formulas preserves their integrity and their nutritional content.

The Daily Protection line packs a powerful punch against environmental free radicals, with an SPF 30 and a healthy boost of antioxidants. The peptides in the mix also stimulate collagen production so skin stays softer, smoother and younger-looking.

# ◈ MD Formulations

MD Formulations was the first line to patent glycolic acid in the use of skincare formulas. This ingredient serves as the cornerstone for MD Formulations products, which are appropriate for all skin types and needs. The company carries an extensive line of formulas, including cleansers, moisturizers, and skin protection. It also offers a full line of body care products. Its products are marketed under the umbrella of Bare Escentuals, Inc., which also offers a mineral makeup line known as Bare Minerals. While the introductory years of the company, started by Diane Richardson in 1976, were rocky at best, Richardson continued to work hard to bring the company into the profitable state she knew was possible. From its humble beginnings in Los Gatos, California, Bare Escentuals (and MD Formulations) is now available at 120-company owned stores in the United States. Its products are also distributed through reputable retailers online. The MD Formulations products have been marketed on QVC and through direct-response infomercials.

Glycolic acid is the key ingredient in most of the MD Formulations products, due to its ability to gently exfoliate the skin without causing irritation. When skin is properly exfoliated, new skin cell growth is promoted for a healthier, younger looking complexion.

MD Formulations products suggest four distinct skincare steps:

❖ Cleanse

❖ Correct

❖ Hydrate

❖ Protect

The cleansers in the MD Formulations line are created to dissolve dirt and exfoliate the surface of the skin for a completely clean complexion. Corrective products are used to address specific skin issues, such as hyper-pigmentation, acne, and the effects of aging. The Continuous Renewal Serum uses the skin cell renewal process to reduce the appearance of fine lines and wrinkles for a younger-looking complexion.

Hydration products are designed to keep the skin soft and supple while using antioxidants to protect the complexion from environmental damage. The Moisture Defense Antioxidant Lotion is used to restore vital moisture and guard against free radical damage that can lead to aging skin. The protection line of MD Formulations products includes sunscreen options, including lip balm and a formula specifically created for sensitive skin.

## ◈ MD FORTE

The maker of MD Forte, Allergan, is a California-based pharmaceutical company that markets a wide range of products including a skincare line. Cosmetic procedures like Botox and a variety of wrinkle fillers are among Allergan's most well known products, and the growing popularity of MD Forte is bringing this product line to the attention of many doctors and clients. However, Allergan purchased MD Forte from Herald Pharmacal about 15 years ago, and since that time, Allergan has introduced many other formulas to the MD Forte lineup.

The base ingredient for all the MD Forte products is glycolic acid, an alpha hydroxy acid that provides a wealth of benefits to the skin. This substance is an exfoliating ingredient that effectively sloughs off dead, dry skin cells, revealing the younger, smoother skin underneath. Alpha hydroxy acids also help the skin retain moisture, which results in a younger complexion.

The product website claims that MD Forte skincare combines the potency of glycolic acid with the process of partial neutralization. This allows for higher concentrations of glycolic acid – and greater potency – without the risk of skin irritation. For sensitive skin that cannot handle exposure to glycolic acid, MD Forte offers a non-AHA product line as well.

MD Forte facial cleansers come in three different strengths to help clients tailor their products to their specific skin types. Level I is typically prescribed to patients who have never used glycolic-acid based products before, or for those who have particularly sensitive skin. Level III is the most potent formula with a 30% glycolic acid base; it is appropriate for all skin types with a doctor's recommendation.

MD Forte renewal lotion products are specifically designed to combat the effects of aging, including the appearance of fine lines and wrinkles. Like the MD Forte facial cleanser, these formulas are graded in terms of potency, allowing the doctor and client to customize the skincare regimen. The renewal line also includes an eye cream with retinol and antioxidants to treat the fine lines and wrinkles that commonly appear in the eye area. It should be noted that the products available through retailers do not offer the same concentrations as those available from a physician.

## ◈ MEG21

Dynamis Skin Science Company is a division of Dynamis Therapeutics, Inc., a pharmaceutical company founded in 1997 by a group of scientists initially specializing in cancer. The company got immediate support from numerous investors, including the Ben Franklin Technology Center and the National Institute of Health. These investors saw great potential for the business and had very high hopes for it. Their confidence was justified when Meg21 was introduced.

Meg21 slows aging by stopping the glycation process and delivering a sufficient dose of amino acids and amino sugars through a liposomal system, allowing the formulas to penetrate the epidermis and get to the root cause of skin flaws like lines, wrinkles, age spots, acne, and more. By delivering these ingredients through the liposomal system, the amino acids and amino sugars in Meg21 break apart and disperse themselves throughout the skin for better and quicker absorption.

## ◈ NEOCUTIS

The origins of Neocutis date back to 2003, when researchers discovered that fetal tissue had the wonderful ability to self-heal without scarring. The company used that technology to develop a line of skincare treatments that utilize Processed Skin Cell Proteins or PSPs in their formulas. The technology was used to effectively treat the following skin disorders:

❖ Acute and chronic wound healing

❖ Psoriasis

❖ Eczema

❖ Vulvodynia

The same cell bank used to produce treatments for these conditions is now also used to produce effective skincare formulas that are only available with a doctor's prescription. Products like the Neocutis Bio-Restorative Skin Cream can be used to fight the effects of aging and as a post-procedural treatment option.

PSPs are the primary ingredients used in all the Neocutis products. These proteins were derived from a one-time fetal donation and are stored in a designated cell bank for future use. The products do not directly use original donated tissues in any way; instead, they use the proteins derived from the cultured skin cells. No further donations will ever be needed in the production of the Neocutis formulas since the cell bank is capable of producing millions of proteins for this purpose.

Neocutis researchers have found that aging skin has many needs similar to those of wounded skin in terms of causing rejuvenation to take place. The growth factors and cytokines found in the PSPs provide the perfect synergistic blend to promote reversal of the environmental damage that led to the aging process in the first place.

One of the best known Neocutis products for cosmaceutical purposes is the Neocutis Bio-Restorative Skin Cream. This formula uses PSPs to reduce the appearance of fine lines and wrinkles and improve skin texture and tone. The Neocutis Lumiere Bio-Restorative Eye Cream combines PSPs with hydrating ingredients like sodium hyaluraonate for brighter, younger looking eyes. In addition to smoothing out fine lines and wrinkles in the eye area, the Lumiere eye cream also reduces the appearance of dark circles and puffiness that are commonly seen during the aging process.

## ◈ NeoStrata Skincare

NeoStrata offers a variety of washes, serums, gels, lotions, cleansers, and creams that transform the skin into a younger and more beautiful version of itself. It combats conditions like acne, fine lines and wrinkles, brown age spots, oily skin, rosacea, discoloration, psoriasis, sagging, eczema, and keratosis pilaris and reveals a healthier appearance underneath. Many of the company's formulas contain either SPF 15 or SPF 20 in order to protect you from the sun's dangerous ultraviolet rays. You'll also be shielded from things like pollution and smoke. Some of the products are specifically designed to treat more targeted areas, like the skin around the eyes. It also offers a product designed for use before and after a procedure—both very crucial times in skin therapy.

Many of the ingredients in the NeoStrata line are drawn from nature and then scientifically enhanced to maximize their power and potency. Containing ingredients like orange peel, primrose, avocado, beeswax, grape, green tea, chamomile, and vitamins E, H, B6, and B3, NeoStrate products are designed to fight acne, improve gmwrinkles, and eliminate imperfections. Many of these products have been created especially for oily skin and therefore also help to prevent and reduce breakouts.

## ◈ Neova Skincare

Neova utilizes a copper peptide therapy complex that is highly effective in halting the signs of aging, because it helps the skin heal itself. It encourages the production and rehabilitation of collagen and elastin and acts almost as an antioxidant.

Neova has products that can be used throughout the day and some that are meant for application at night. Several of the formulas are based on retinol. There are treatments designed specifically for the eyes (suitable for the sensitive skin in that area) and many of the formulas take into account skin sensitivities or allergies. Neova offers a microdermabrasion scrub, as well as a selection of shampoos, conditioners, follicle sprays, and even eyelash conditioners.

## ◈ Nia24 Skincare

Not too long ago, Myron and Elaine Jacobson—both professors at the University of Arizona College of

Pharmacy and with more than a quarter century of biomedical experience each—were doing intense research on niacin. During their studies, they discovered that it had an amazing effect on human skin. They founded Niadyne, Inc., officially based in North Carolina, and introduced Nia24, a line based entirely around this ingredient.

The Nia24 products come in all shapes, sizes, and consistencies and are especially designed to treat existing sun damage and to protect the skin from future damage. The formulas come in scrubs, creams, serums, lotions, sunscreen, moisturizers, and cleansers. In addition, Nia24 includes products that target problem areas like the eyes. This skincare line is unique because of the way it restores and shields the skin both inside and out. Products are applied topically, but through a slow, thorough, continuous release of ingredients, Nia24 products penetrate deep into your skin tissue.

## ◈ Nuxe Paris

Nuxe Paris was established in Paris, France in 1957 by an educated and well-trained pharmacist. The company is known for the powerful formulas it produces and for the healthy, natural ingredients it uses to make them. Its anti-aging products in particular are known for their potency.

The formulas are suitable for all skin types, for both men and women, and address a range of skin conditions. Nuxe Paris also has a cosmaceutical line of cosmetics for women.

## ◈ Obagi

Obagi Medical Products is a company that offers pharmaceutical-grade skincare options through physicians and medical spas. However, the company also offers a line of non-prescription products available through some online retailers.

Obagi officially began operations under this name in 1997, although the initial product line known as the Obagi Nu-Derm System was introduced in 1988. Since that time, the company has continued to grow, expanding its product line to even more clinically-proven skin systems that can be effectively used by dermatologists, plastic surgeons, and other aesthetic professionals. The company is headquartered in Long Beach, California, but its reputation has now spread across the globe.

Ingredients used in Obagi products are pharmaceutical grade and can address skin issues from pigmentation problems to photo damage. Obagi is known for its development of the Blue Peel, which can be used in conjunction with the Obagi Nu-Derm system to produce a complete skin transformation. This peel utilizes alpha hydroxy acids, which have been proven to exfoliate the skin and promote skin cell renewal. The AHAs can be adjusted in terms of strength to address a host of skin needs.

Obagi offers a line of vitamin C-based products, which have been shown to brighten skin tone and stimulate collagen production for more supple skin. Vitamin C is also an effective antioxidant that protects the skin from free radical damage and makes the skin look younger for longer.

The Obagi products are sold in systems, ensuring that individuals get the full benefit of its formulas working together for best results. However, customers can also purchase non-prescription products separately through online retailers if they prefer.

One customer favorite is the Obagi Nu-Derm Foaming Gel, which offers the deep cleansing that oily and normal skin types require. Ingredients like Aloe Vera are included in the formula to soothe skin after cleansing and prevent irritation. The Obagi Nu-Derm Toner is designed to be used after the foaming gel to help readjust the skin's pH and allow increased penetration from the rest of the formulas in the system.

## ◈ OLE HENRIKSEN

Often referred to as the "facialist to the stars," Ole Henriksen has designed an array of natural skincare products that use pure, highly effective ingredients. When developing a new product, Ole Henriksen considers how the product interacts with the skin. He then combines the new formulation, which typically includes exotic and effective ingredients, with the current portfolio of soothing, hydrating, retexturizing, and renewing ingredients already used in the Ole Henriksen line of skincare products.

The complete line is safe and effective for nearly every skin types.

## ◈ PANGEA ORGANICS

All of the products of Pangea Organics are naturally derived, and all ingredients in the skincare line are organic and pure; there are no petro-chemicals, parabens, GMOs, or synthetic ingredients. They also never include petroleum-based ingredients, sulfates, detergents, or artificial colors or fragrances.

Based in Boulder, Colorado, Pangea Organics was founded on the principle of creating a sustainable future through the use of organic skincare and body care products. All products in the Pangea Organics skincare line are designed to help—not harm—people through all the stages of their lives.

Pangea Organic products are therapeutic for both the mind and the body, and they are beneficial and safe, both for people and the planet. The skincare products have been created for nearly any type of skin at any stage in life.

Pangea Organics practices sustainable agriculture and culture, from fair trade and sourcing to organic farming and the use of renewable, recyclable resources.

## ◈ PCA SKIN

PCA Skincare was first started in 1990, by licensed aesthetician Margaret Ancira. In 2006, PCA Skin added Jennifer Linder, M.D., to its staff. Dr. Linder is a board-certified dermatologist who guides product development and clinical trials for PCA Skincare.

Today, under the guidance of CEO Richard Linder, PCA Skincare has expanded to offer a wide line of skincare products. This company has complete lines for daily care at home, as well as a variety of professional treatments. It also carries a full line of men's skincare products.

The primary ingredients used in PCA Skincare include:

❖ Alpha Hydroxy Acids (AHAs)

❖ Antioxidants

❖ Substances for Pigment Control

❖ Substances for Acne Control

❖ Peptides

According to many PCA Skincare reviews, AHAs are effective in exfoliating the skin, leaving it softer and smoother after treatment. These ingredients also address skin needs at the cellular level, by promoting skin cell renewal that effectively turns back the clock on the complexion. Antioxidants fight the effects of environmental free radicals, such as pollution and the UV rays from the sun, to prevent skin damage.

Pigment control is achieved through active ingredients like hydroquinone and Kojic acid, which are both proven skin lighteners. PCA Skincare keeps acne at bay through bacteria busting ingredients like benzoyl peroxide, salicylic acid, and sulfur,

Peptides are a relative newcomer to the anti-aging scene, and they have been proven to reduce the appearance of fine lines and wrinkles through a number of methods. PCA Skin products include Acetyl Hexapeptide-3 and Palmitoyl Oligopeptide.

The PCA pHaze 5 Nutrient Toner is considered one of the best in its category for nourishing the skin and preparing it for further treatment. This formula includes a potent punch of vitamins and AHAs. The PCA pHaze 1 Facial Wash uses AHAs in a gentle formula that thoroughly cleanses even as it calms the skin.

## ◈ PEVONIA

Spas using Pevonia treatments can be found around the globe, including at a number of locations in the United States. Pevonia Botanica technicians are highly trained in the use of its products, which ensures an optimal experience for the consumer.

Pevonia packs its products with high-quality, science-based ingredients like vitamin C, retinol and hyaluronic acid. Hyaluronic acid is an effective substance for hydrating skin from the inside out, for reversing the early signs of aging, and for moisturizing dry skin. All Pevonia formulas are non-comedogenic and contain no artificial fragrances or colors.

The line includes many best-seller products, including the Age-Defying Marine Collagen Cream and a variety of exfoliating cleansers. The collagen cream is touted as both a moisturizer and an anti-aging treatment that contains marine collagen, hyaluronic acid, and squalane. Titanium dioxide, another ingredient, offers sun block to protect the skin while it treats the damage that has already been done.

The Gentle Exfoliating Cleanser removes layers of dirt and dead skin cells for a softer, smoother complexion. Jojoba beads give this formula a grainy texture that cleanses without drying skin. This Pevonia product also works to prevent clogged pores.

## ◈ Peter Thomas Roth

Peter Thomas Roth used his family's background to develop a skincare line that had a clinical focus. His research and development is focused on formulas that effectively treat a host of skincare needs, while offering the necessary protection to prevent further damage. In 1993, Roth founded his company by creating soothing skincare products containing the minerals and mud found in the thermal springs around his home in Hungary. Roth combined forces with his friend and skincare creator, June Jacobs, to improve the products by adding top quality ingredients that utilized the latest science. By combining traditional healing substances with the latest scientific technology, he was able to create results-based skincare formulas that quickly became popular with the general public.

Peter Thomas Roth offers an extensive skincare line. This company is well known for cleansers and exfoliating formulas that effectively remove dead, dry skin cells and dirt for a cleaner, clearer complexion. Exfoliating products offer unique Botanical Buffing Beads in combination with naturally exfoliating ingredients like salicylic acid. Peter Thomas Roth eye cream removes puffiness around the eyes.

Peter Thomas Roth is also known for its sun protection products, which include both mineral and chemical-based formulas. Most of the sun care options offer an SPF 30, although the Instant Mineral formula recommended by the Skin Cancer Foundation provides an SPF 45 for maximum protection. A sunless tanning product, it allows users to get full sun protection and still flaunt a healthy glow all year long.

## ❖ Philip B Skincare

Philip B has a long history as the preeminent hair care expert to the Hollywood crowd. Philip B went in search of the finest hair care products the world had to offer, but after searching meticulously through the most well-known and luxurious brands, he was disappointed with the predictable blends of harsh chemicals and cheap ingredients. He knew firsthand the power of natural botanicals, so working in his own kitchen he began to create custom blends packed with powerful treatments elements.

The result of this labor of love was the Philip B Rejuvenating Oil, a treatment oil fine enough to penetrate the hair shaft without leaving behind a sticky residue. From that one product, the Philip B family of treatment options was born. The Hollywood A-Listers, social elite, and even royalty are counted among the brand's loyal customers. Today, the line has expanded to include a wide variety of nourishing treatment options, yet the Rejuvenating Oil still remains the most recognized product of all.

Today, Philip B remains directly involved in every aspect of the product line to ensure that quality standards are maintained and effectiveness is ensured.

## ◈ Replenix

The Replenix skincare line is the brainchild of Topix Pharmaceuticals, a New York-based company founded in 1981 by Stanley Shaffer. Today, Shaffer's son Burt is the company's president and owner. He carries on the tradition of creating effective skincare and other personal hygiene products, most of which are available by prescription only.

The company conducts research and development, production, and testing of all of its products from a state-of-the-art, FDA-approved facility in New York. In addition to the Replenix brand, Topix is also known for its Citrix and Glycolix Elite brands.

Today, Replenix is available through spas, high-end stores, and online retailers. While customers cannot purchase products directly from the Topix website, they can find extensive information about the company's formulas so they can make informed decisions about Replenix products prior to making a purchase.

The primary, most effective ingredient in all Replenix formulas is polyphenol, which is extracted from green tea. The benefits of polyphenol have been well documented, both for its health and cosmetic advantages.

Green tea reduces damage from sun exposure by combating environmental free radicals found in harmful UV rays. Because green tea extracts do not actually block UV rays, the combination of polyphenols with UV blocking ingredients is particularly effective.

In addition to polyphenols and the potent sun blocking ingredients found in all the Replenix formulas, products may also contain effective anti-aging ingredients like hyaluronic acid, which hydrates skin from the inside out to create a smoother, younger appearance. Retinol, a derivative of vitamin A has also been shown to be effective in reducing the appearance of fine lines and is included in the All-trans-Retinol Smoothing Serum.

While Replenix offers a relatively small skincare line, there are products to address a variety of skin concerns, including cleansers, exfoliating products and serums to hydrate the skin and target specific concerns like aging, sun damage, or dry skin.

## ◈ SkinMedica

Dr. Fitzpatrick used his own knowledge and personal experiences from his dermatology practice when creating the SkinMedica product line. When the pharmaceutical products developed a large and loyal following in the medical community, Dr. Fitzpatrick decided to make his formulas available to the general public as well. The company now offers both a professional and a personal line of skincare products to address the full gamut of skincare needs.

SkinMedica uses ingredients like vitamins E, C and A. Retinol, a derivative of vitamin A, is an effective skin exfoliator and has been used in skincare lines to address concerns from acne to aging. The company also uses a patented combination of growth factors, soluble collagen and matrix proteins to effectively reduce the appearance of fine lines and wrinkles and promote more firmness and elasticity in aging skin. The antioxidants used in the products protect the skin from environmental free radical damage to prevent the signs of aging and keep skin soft and supple for as long as possible.

SkinMedica offers products to cleanse and tone the skin, as well as a range of formulas to address specific skin needs. The Age Defense line is probably the largest for SkinMedica, with complexes and serums designed to address the specific concerns of aging like loss of collagen and elastin, sun damage, and the appearance of fine lines and wrinkles. Products work on a variety of concerns, with special formulas designed for problem areas like the eyes and lips.

The TNS Essential Serum combines two active formulas that work together to produce a more youthful complexion. Ingredients like proteins, antioxidants, and peptides work synergistically to reduce the signs of aging. The SkinMedica Retinol Complex provides three forms of vitamin A to offer a powerful punch of exfoliation and skin regeneration to improve skin texture and tone.

## ◈ SOMME INSTITUTE

Armed with some of the best research and development laboratories from around the globe, the Somme Institute has developed and patented technology called MDT5 — or Molecular Dispersion Technology.

MDT5 can penetrate the deepest layers of skin to completely change its texture and alter its overall appearance and radiance. This non-prescription formula combines high concentrations of five vitamins — A, C, E, B3 and B5 — that penetrate the skin's innermost layers.

The technology behind the Somme Institute's MDT5 allows these vitamins to penetrate the skin without oxidizing and without losing their potency once they are exposed to air and light.

Using the MDT5 technology, the Somme Institute has developed a highly effective skincare regimen to be used twice daily. It involves the products Transport, Serum, and A-Bomb.

**Transport** — Transport, which is infused with AHA/BHA, is designed to exfoliate dead skin cells and unclog blocked pores. Transport makes it possible for key vitamins to be delivered deep into the skin, speeding up cell renewal and improving skin hydration and resiliency.

**Serum**—Serum features an advanced, potent form of vitamin C, which works along with MDT5 to strengthen the skin's elasticity and smooth the appearance of fine lines and wrinkles.

**A-Bomb**—A-Bomb quickly penetrates the deepest layers of the skin with a high concentration of vitamins A and E; this vitamin duo, along with the MDT5 technology, restores cell function, softens lines, and targets problem areas.

The Somme Institute regimen, which calls for the MDT5 trio to be used in concert with the Nourishing Cleanser and the Double Defense:

❖ Treats moderate to severe acne

❖ Reduces the appearance of fine lines and wrinkles

❖ Reverses sun damage and lightens brown spots

❖ Dramatically improves skin's texture, tone, and clarity

The Somme Institute recommends supplementing the MDT5 line with its Nourishing Cleanser and its Double Defense, which has an SPF 30. The cleanser is designed to prepare the skin for the MDT5 core treatment, while the Double Defense is designed to hydrate and protect the skin from the damaging effects of the sun.

## ◈ Sothys

Sothys got its start more than 60 years ago, with a professional brand used in high-end institutes, spas, and at home. Professional formulas are designed to be used with massage techniques to produce the best results. Home care products are meant to supplement and prolong the results of spa treatments over a longer period of time.

Sothys' anti-aging formulas incorporate proven ingredients like peptides and hyaluronic acid that hydrate skin from the inside out and promote collagen production for smoother, younger skin. The corrective line of Sothys products includes marine extracts and antioxidants that support skin health and vitality while targeting a variety of specific skin issues.

Sothys product line is organized on the company website into a variety of categories that help consumers find formulas that will meet their needs. Because Sothys believes that properly cleansed skin responds much better to treatment, there is a great deal of emphasis placed on highly effective cleansers, exfoliators, and moisturizers.

Deep cleansing products incorporate astringents and clarifying substances that effectively eliminate all impurities while their standard cleansers use soothing ingredients like Shea butter and sweet almond oil for gentle cleansing. Sothys products are targeted to maintain skin that has been properly treated, moisturize dry skin, and treat specific concerns. There is also a skincare line designed just for men.

## ◈ YONKA

Yonka skincare began with three botanist brothers from France: Cecile, Ernst, and Charles Muhlethaler. In 1957, these men created the Multaler Laboratories, where they worked with doctors and scientists to develop formulas using Quintessence, a unique blend of five essential oils from the Mediterranean that would become the basis for their first Yonka skincare line. The brothers combined these essential oils with other ingredients found in plants and the sea to produce skincare formulas that promoted skin health, and at the same time, produced stellar aesthetic results.

The success of the Yonka products resulted in a rapidly growing company that opened subsidiaries in the United States, Great Britain, and Switzerland by the turn of the century. In 2003, Yonka opened its own extensive spa on the Left Bank of Paris, which provides a wealth of treatment options to customers.

Yonka skincare uses four botanical therapies in their product lines:

❖ Aromatherapy through essential oils designed to heal, relax, and invigorate

❖ Phytotherapy that uses plants to promote health and healing

❖ Marine therapy that takes ingredients from the sea to nourish the skin

❖ Fruit acid therapy that provides gentle exfoliation and promotes skin cell renewal

Today, more than 130 plants are combined with the original five essential oils to produce potent formulas that treat skin without irritating it.

# CONCLUSION

A s you have learned in this book, it is never too early to start pampering your skin. Early prevention and pro-active intervention can really make a difference in the way your skin looks at the age you are now, and it paves the way for how your skin will look and feel when it begins to age.

Committing to a consistent, well-planned skin care regimen using top of the line products geared to meet the needs of your particular skin type is your best ally in keeping your skin looking young, feeling fresh, and staying blemish-free.

If you have skin issues now, like acne, rosacea, psoriasis, early onset aging, or even skin cancers, there is help available. By connecting with a good dermatologist, esthetician, or other skin care specialist, you are, in essence, buying insurance against the pre-mature aging that these skin damaging conditions can cause. Professionals can help you establish a skin care plan that is best for your skin type and recommend the proper treatments and products to address existing issues. Through their careful intervention and your home use of the appropriate products, these issues can be resolved and a prescribed course of action can be established to keep them under control.

It's never too early to start a skin care regime, and it is never too late. Whether you're still in your teens or a Baby Boomer well into your retirement years, there are products and programs that will help you stop the clock and refresh the skin you're in. Make a few changes today, and just see where tomorrow takes you.

# REFERENCES

Bailey, A.J. (2001, May 31). *Molecular mechanisms of ageing in connective tissues.*

PubMed. 7, pp. 735–755.

Benedetto, AV. (1998, Jan–Feb). *The environment and skin aging.* 1, pp. 129–139.

Darr, D. Dunston, S., Faust, H., Pinnell, S. (1996, July) *Effectiveness of antioxidants (vitamin C and E) with and without sunscreens as topical photoprotectants.* 4, pp. 264–268.

Denese, A. M.D., Ph.D, (2005) *Younger skin in 8 weeks.* New York, N.Y.: Penguin Group.

Dreher, F. & Maibach, H. (2001) *Protective effects of topical antioxidants in humans.* PubMed, 29, pp. 157–164.

Elson, ML. (1995–1998) *Topical Phytonadione (vitamin K) in the treatment of actinic and traumatic purpura.* Cosmetic Dermatology, 12, pp. 25–27.

Goldberg, D.J. M.D. & Herriott, E.M. (2003). *The definitive guide to anti-aging skin care.* Herndon, VA., Capital Books, Inc.

Guttman, C. (2002, September 1) *Studies demonstrate value of procollagen fragment Pal–TTKS.* Dermatological Times. 23, p. 9.

Jepson, S., M.D. (2008). *7 Ways to look younger without undergoing "the knife".* Murray, Utah. (SSP).

Katina, SK., Matsui, MS., Elmets, CA., & Mukhtar H. (1999, Feb) *Polyphenolic antioxidant (-)-epigallocatechin-3-gallate from green tea reduces UVB-induced inflammatory*

*responses and infiltration of leukocytes in human skin.*
PubMed, 2, pp.148–153.

Landau M.(2005, Dec. 17) *Advances in deep chemical peels.*
PubMed, 6, pp. 438–441.

Laugier, JP. et al. (2000) *Topical hyaluronidase decreases
hyaluronic acid and CD44 in human skin and in reconstituted
human epidermis: evidence that hyaluronidase can permeate the
stratum corneum.* British Journal of Dermatology 142, pp.
226–233.

Lou WW; Quintana AT; Geronemus RG; Grossman MC
(1999 Dec. 25). *Effects of topical vitamin K and retinol on laser-
induced purpura on nonlesional skin.* Dermatologic Surgery
12, pp. 942–944.

Lupo, MP. (2001). *Antioxidants and vitamins in cosmetics.*
Clinical Dermatology. 19, pp. 467–473.

McVean, M. & Liebler, DC.(1997, August 18) *Inhibition of
UVB induced DNA photodamage in mouse epidermis by
topically applied alpha-tocopherol.* PubMed, 8, pp. 1617–1622.

Oikarinen A. (1994, April 10) *Aging of the skin connective
tissue: how to measure the biochemical and mechanical
properties of aging dermis.* Photodermatology,
Photoimmunology and Photomedicine, 2, pp. 47–52.

Rokhsar, CK., Lee, S., & Fitzpatrick RE. (2005, September)
*Review of Photorejuvenation: Devices, Cosmeceuticals, or Both.*
Dermatologic Surgery. Part 2, 31, p. 9.

Shah, NS. Et al. (2002 August). *The effects of topical vitamin K
on bruising after laser treatment.* Journal of the American
Academy of Dermatology. 47, pp. 241–244.

Stratigos, AJ. & Katsambas, AD. (2005) *The role of topical retinoids in the treatment of photoaging.* PubMed. 8, pp. 1061–72.

Whang, S. (1990) *Reverse aging.* Miami, Fl. (SSP).

www.ingramcontent.com/pod-product-compliance
Lightning Source LLC
Chambersburg PA
CBHW060241290526
45789CB00001B/136